Plato's Press

CHICAGO, ILLINOIS

THE LIBRARY
OF Congress HAS
CATALOGUED THIS TEXT AS FOLLOWS
Registration: XXX

Volume 1
HEALTHCARE
Ethics Consultant's
HANDBOOK

A Comprehensive Guide to Ethical Decision-Making in Clinical Practice

Description: Electronic File (eService)
Copyright: Jeffrey Wallace Bulger
Date of Creation: xx/xx/2024
Authorship: Jeffrey Wallace Bulger
Rights and Permissions: Jeffrey Wallace Bulger

ISBN 978-1-62252-029-9
9 781622 520299

Volume 1
HEALTHCARE
Ethics Consultant's
HANDBOOK

A Comprehensive Guide to Ethical Decision-Making in Clinical Practice

---

Book Description

Volume 1 of the Healthcare Ethics Handbook Series
Healthcare professionals face complex ethical issues daily, demanding thoughtful and structured responses. *Volume 1 — Healthcare Ethics Consultant's Handbook: A Comprehensive Guide to Ethical Decision-Making in Clinical Practice*, the first in a three-volume series, provides a foundational framework for ethics consultants and healthcare professionals. This volume equips readers with practical strategies and methodologies for navigating ethical challenges, laying the groundwork for further discussions in Volumes 2 and 3.

Key Features:

- **Foundations of Medical Ethics Consultation**: Explore the evolution and critical role of ethics consultation in patient care.
- **Core Principles of Bioethics**: Understand autonomy, beneficence, nonmaleficence, and justice.
- **The Ethics Consultation Process**: Step-by-step guidance from initiation to documentation.
- **Practical Skills for Ethics Consultants**: Enhance communication, mediation, and cultural competence.

- **Special Topics in Medical Ethics**: Explore issues like end-of-life care, informed consent, and research ethics.
- **Education and Professional Development**: Strategies for continuous growth.
- **Practical Tools and Resources**: Utilize templates for effective communication and documentation.
- **Real-World Case Studies**: Learn from ethical complexities.
- **Review Questions and Further Readings**: Reinforce knowledge.

About the Series:

The *Healthcare Ethics Handbook Series* is a three-volume resource for navigating ethical challenges in healthcare. Volume 1 focuses on ethical decision-making and clinical consultation, Volume 2 emphasizes bioethics leadership, and Volume 3 addresses 60 clinical ethics topics. The series grounds readers in the core bioethical principles, equipping them for leadership.

About the Author:

Dr. Jeffrey W. Bulger brings both academic and practical expertise to medical ethics. His recent book, *Bioethics: Passing the Boards, Providing Patient Care, and Beyond*, published by Oxford University Press, reflects his dedication to guiding healthcare professionals through ethical challenges.

***

Table of Contents

Volume 1

HEALTHCARE Ethics Consultant's HANDBOOK

A Comprehensive Guide to Ethical Decision-Making in Clinical Practice

---

Part I: Foundations of Medical Ethics Consultation

Introduction to Medical Ethics Consultation

In the intricate and ever-evolving realm of healthcare, ethical dilemmas are inevitable and constantly shifting in complexity. As an aspiring or experienced clinical ethicist, you stand at the crossroads of medicine, morality, and law, guiding patients, families, and healthcare providers through decisions that often carry profound implications. Medical ethics consultation is not merely a component of contemporary healthcare—it is an integral pillar that ensures decisions are made thoughtfully, compassionately, and in alignment with ethical principles, institutional policies, and legal mandates.

This section serves as your gateway into the foundational concepts of medical ethics consultation. We will delve into the dynamic nature of medical standards of care and explore the four core bioethical principles that underpin ethical decision-making in healthcare. Through the compelling case study of Mr. Thompson, you will witness how these principles are applied in real-world scenarios, setting the stage for a deeper exploration of ethics consultation methodologies in the sections that follow.

Understanding Medical Ethics Consultation

The Role and Importance in Healthcare

Imagine being part of a healthcare team faced with a decision that has no clear right or wrong answer—a situation where medical facts intertwine with personal goals, values, and priorities, medical standards of care, institutional policies, and legal considerations. Medical ethics consultation emerges as a vital resource in such moments, providing a structured forum for open dialogue. It helps clarify values, address moral distress, and facilitate consensus among all parties involved. As an ethics consultant, you play a pivotal role in ensuring that patient care decisions are made thoughtfully, respecting the dignity and rights of patients while balancing the perspectives of families and healthcare providers.

By integrating ethical considerations into clinical practice, ethics consultations not only enhance the quality of care but also promotes a culture of ethical awareness within healthcare institutions. They serve as a reminder that medicine is not just about curing diseases but also about caring for people in a manner that honors their reasonable goals, values, and priorities.

Medical Standards of Care

Definition and Misconceptions

The term "medical standards of care" may often suggest rigid protocols governing every aspect of treatment. However, these standards are more nuanced and fluid. They refer to the level and type of care that a reasonably competent healthcare professional, with similar training and in comparable circumstances, would provide. Medical standards of care are shaped by evidence-based, peer-reviewed practices and the consensus of the medical profession. While not fixed directives, these standards evolve alongside advancements in medical research, technology, and shifting societal values. As ethical and legal benchmarks, they help assess the appropriateness of medical interventions, ensuring high-quality care and professional accountability.

The Importance of Staying Current

Understanding the fluidity of these standards is crucial. A treatment once deemed standard a decade ago may now be outdated due to new research findings. As an ethics consultant, it is essential to remain informed about these developments to provide guidance that aligns with the best current practices, while also considering the unique circumstances of each case. For example, a once-standard invasive surgery may now be replaced by minimally invasive procedures as research and technology advance.

Contextual Application of Standards

Medical standards of care are dynamic, continuously shaped by advancements in research that introduce new treatments and therapies, thus shifting what constitutes appropriate care. Moreover, regional differences, resource availability, and specific patient populations can significantly impact how these standards are applied. For instance, a treatment easily accessible in a large, well-equipped urban hospital might not be feasible in a rural setting with limited resources. As an ethics consultant, it's important to take these contextual factors into account when offering guidance.

A Fluid and Context-Dependent Framework

Recognizing that medical standards of care are not fixed but instead fluid and context-dependent is vital to effective ethics consultation. For example, in end-of-life care, the standard of care may shift from aggressive treatment to comfort-focused palliative care based on the patient's condition and expressed wishes. This flexibility requires careful consideration of the patient's reasonable goals, values, and priorities. By doing so, you help ensure that care decisions are ethically sound, medically appropriate, and aligned with current standards.

The Four Bioethical Principles

Ethical decision-making in healthcare is guided by four core bioethical principles that serve as the foundation for your practice:

1. **Patient Autonomy** (Informed Consent): Respecting the patient's right to make informed decisions about their treatment options. This involves ensuring the patient (or their surrogate) comprehends their diagnosis, prognosis, all viable treatment options (including the option to decline treatment), and the associated risks and benefits. Consent must be given voluntarily, without coercion, and align with the patient's reasonable goals, values, and priorities, while adhering to medical standards of care, institutional policies, and legal requirements. The consent should be clearly communicated and formally documented in the medical records. Informed consent is an ongoing process that must be revisited as the patient's condition evolves or as new treatment options emerge.
2. **Practitioner Beneficence** (Maximizing Benefits): Providing treatment options that promote the patient's well-being, as determined by the patient's reasonable goals, values, and priorities. These options must also be within the boundaries of medical standards of care, institutional policies, and legal requirements, ensuring that interventions act in the patient's best interest while adhering to established protocols. Practitioners should actively seek to identify treatment options that provide the most benefit, even when they are less conventional, as long as they remain within medical standards of care.
3. **Practitioner Nonmaleficence** (Minimizing Burdens): Avoiding treatment options that cause unnecessary harm or suffering to the patient, ensuring that harm is minimized by considering the patient's reasonable goals, values, and priorities. Any decisions must conform to medical standards of care, institutional policies, and legal mandates to ensure both ethical soundness and professional accountability. Practitioners must balance the

principles of beneficence and nonmaleficence, as treatments intended to benefit the patient can also carry risks of harm, which must be minimized.

4. **Public Justice** (Ensuring Fairness): Public Justice requires adherence to medical standards of care, institutional policies, and state and federal laws to ensure fair and equitable treatment for all patients within the healthcare system. This includes complying with all policies and regulations that mandate the fair distribution of care and resources, free from bias or favoritism, and aligning decisions with the broader responsibilities of the healthcare community. Public Justice also involves ensuring that vulnerable populations receive equitable care and that healthcare disparities are actively addressed.

These principles provide a framework for evaluating and guiding ethical decisions, helping balance individual patient needs with professional responsibilities and societal considerations. They are interrelated and often must be weighed against each other to arrive at the most ethical course of action.

Decisional Capacity

Definition

Decisional capacity is essential for respecting Patient Autonomy, as it determines a patient's ability to participate meaningfully in the informed consent process. It means that a patient (or their surrogate) can fulfill the conditions necessary for informed consent as outlined under Patient Autonomy.

Key Components of Decisional Capacity

1. **Understanding:** The patient (or their surrogate) must have the capacity to comprehend the medical information related to their condition and proposed treatment options. This includes a clear grasp of their diagnosis, prognosis, and all viable treatment options, including the option to decline treatment.

2. **Appreciation:** The patient (or their surrogate) must understand the potential outcomes of consenting to or declining treatment,

including the benefits and risks associated with each option. This self-awareness ensures they can weigh how each decision impacts their personal circumstances and aligns with their reasonable goals, values, and priorities.

3. **Reasoning:** The patient (or their surrogate) must logically evaluate the risks and benefits of various treatment options and their short-term and long-term implications. They should consider how each option aligns with their reasonable goals, values, and priorities. This evaluation must also adhere to medical standards of care, institutional policies, and legal regulations.
4. **Communication:** The patient (or their surrogate) must clearly convey their decision to the healthcare team. Effective communication ensures that the patient's informed consent is properly documented in the patient's medical record.

Assessment of Decisional Capacity

Healthcare providers often utilize standardized assessment tools that evaluate these key components. Tools specifically designed for this purpose include:

- **MacArthur Competence Assessment Tool for Treatment (MacCAT-T):** A structured interview assessing a patient's capacity to make informed treatment decisions.
- **Aid to Capacity Evaluation (ACE):** A practical tool for clinicians to evaluate decision-making capacity at the bedside.
- **Capacity to Consent to Treatment Instrument (CCTI):** Uses clinical scenarios to assess understanding and reasoning regarding treatment choices.
- **Understanding Treatment Disclosure (UTD):** Measures a patient's comprehension of information provided during the informed consent process.

Integrating these tools into clinical practice upholds ethical standards and legal requirements, ensuring that informed consent is valid and that patient autonomy is respected.

Who Determines Decisional Capacity

In a medical setting, decisional capacity is usually assessed by the primary practitioner responsible for the patient's care, such as the attending physician. Depending on the complexity of the situation, other members of the healthcare team may be involved as consultants in the assessment, including:

- **Psychiatrists or Psychologists:** When mental health issues may affect capacity.
- **Neurologists:** If neurological conditions could impair decision-making abilities.
- **Clinical Ethicists:** For complex ethical considerations.
- **Social Workers or Nurses:** To provide additional insights into the patient's social and cognitive functioning.

While assessing decisional capacity is primarily a clinical judgment, consultation with specialists is important when mental health disorders, cognitive impairments, or other complicating factors are present.

When a Patient Lacks Decisional Capacity

When a patient is deemed to lack decisional capacity, the responsibility for making healthcare decisions shifts to a surrogate decision-maker. This surrogate acts on the patient's behalf, guided by a legal and ethical framework designed to honor the patient's autonomy and ensure their well-being. The surrogate's decisions must align with the patient's known reasonable goals, values, and priorities, adhering to medical standards of care, institutional policies, and legal requirements. In situations where the patient's specific preferences are unknown, the surrogate should act in the patient's best interests, employing the reasonable person standard, which considers what a reasonable person would decide under similar circumstances.

Advance directives play a crucial role in guiding surrogate decision-making. These legal documents enable patients to outline their future healthcare preferences in the event they become unable to communicate their decisions. The two primary forms of advance directives are the Living Will and the Durable Power of Attorney for Healthcare.

A Living Will allows patients to specify their preferences for certain medical treatments if they become incapacitated, particularly concerning end-of-life care. Commonly, it addresses the use of life-sustaining interventions such as mechanical ventilation, resuscitation efforts like CPR, and artificial nutrition and hydration. The living will takes precedence over surrogate decisions because it directly reflects the patient's expressed wishes. Healthcare providers are legally obligated to follow the directives specified in a valid living will, and the surrogate's role becomes one of ensuring these wishes are honored.

On the other hand, a Durable Power of Attorney for Healthcare permits a patient to appoint a trusted individual—a healthcare proxy or agent—to make healthcare decisions on their behalf. The term "durable" signifies that this authority remains effective even if the patient becomes incapacitated, distinguishing it from non-durable powers of attorney that become invalid upon the individual's incapacitation. Typically, the durable power of attorney for healthcare becomes active once the patient is deemed to lack decisional capacity, though some documents may specify immediate activation that continues regardless of the patient's capacity status.

The healthcare proxy has broad authority to make decisions that align with the patient's reasonable goals, values, and priorities as situations arise. However, if a living will exists, the proxy must respect the directives outlined in it. Their authority primarily covers areas not specified in the living will, ensuring that all decisions remain consistent with the patient's wishes.

It's important to note that non-durable powers of attorney, usually associated with financial matters, do not grant authority for decisions after the loss of decisional capacity. These documents become invalid once the individual becomes incapacitated and are not applicable in medical decision-making contexts.

When a surrogate makes decisions for an incapacitated patient, they are expected to apply the principle of substituted judgment. This approach means the surrogate should make choices based on what the patient would have decided if they were capable, using the patient's known values, preferences, and previously expressed wishes as a guide. The goal is to preserve the patient's autonomy by aligning decisions with their established goals, values, and priorities.

In cases where the patient's specific wishes are unknown and cannot be reasonably inferred, the surrogate must rely on the best interest standard. This involves carefully weighing the potential benefits and burdens of each treatment option to determine what would most enhance the patient's overall well-being and quality of life. Factors such as the patient's comfort, dignity, and the likelihood of regaining function or awareness are critical considerations. The surrogate bears the ethical responsibility to make choices that a reasonable person would consider optimal under similar circumstances, always aiming to promote the patient's best interests.

In the absence of a designated healthcare proxy or a living will, state laws typically provide a default hierarchy of surrogate decision-makers. This hierarchy can vary by jurisdiction but often starts with a court-appointed guardian, followed by the patient's spouse or domestic partner, adult children, parents, adult siblings, and then other relatives or close friends who have an established relationship with the patient and are familiar with their values. Healthcare providers should be well-versed in local laws and institutional policies regarding surrogate decision-making to ensure compliance and proper guidance.

Legal considerations are paramount in surrogate decision-making. Laws governing advance directives and surrogate decision-making can differ significantly by state or country, so consultation with legal counsel or reference to institutional policies is advisable for specific guidance. It's essential that all decisions comply with relevant legal requirements to uphold the patient's rights and maintain the ethical standards of care. Thorough documentation of all decisions and the rationale behind them in the patient's medical record is crucial for legal accountability and transparency.

Advance directives serve as a foundational element in respecting patient autonomy. By preparing these documents, patients can maintain control over their healthcare decisions, provide clear guidance to surrogates and healthcare providers, and alleviate the emotional burden on family members who might otherwise face difficult decisions without guidance.

Understanding and honoring advance directives, along with the principles of surrogate decision-making, are integral components of ethical healthcare practice. By adhering to the legal and ethical frameworks outlined, healthcare providers can ensure they respect the patient's autonomy, promote their well-being, and uphold professional and legal standards.

While assessing and involving surrogate decision-makers, it's important to recognize that decisional capacity is task-specific and time-sensitive. A patient's capacity can vary over time due to factors like delirium, medication effects, or fatigue, necessitating periodic reassessment. Healthcare providers should always begin with the presumption that the patient has capacity unless there is clear evidence to the contrary.

Efforts should be made to maximize patient participation in decision-making whenever possible. This can involve employing supportive measures such as using simple language, visual aids, or involving interpreters to enhance understanding. Providing a quiet and comfortable environment can also help the patient focus and better comprehend information.

In complex cases, adopting a multidisciplinary approach can provide a more comprehensive assessment and support system. Involving ethics committees or consulting with specialists can be beneficial when significant disagreements or ethical dilemmas arise. Throughout this process, the goal is to maintain as much patient autonomy as possible, using the least restrictive interventions.

Healthcare providers must ensure that all assessments and decisions comply with medical standards of care and ethical guidelines, following institutional protocols and being mindful of state and federal laws regarding informed consent and decision-making capacity. Thorough documentation of the assessment process, findings, and rationale in the patient's medical record is essential for accountability and continuity of care.

By carefully considering these factors, healthcare providers can make informed, ethical, and legally sound decisions regarding a patient's ability to participate in their own care. This approach not only supports individual patient care but also highlights the vital interplay between ethical principles and legal mandates in healthcare decision-making.

Applying Bioethical Principles: The Case of Mr. Thompson

In the complex and emotionally charged environment of healthcare, the real-world application of ethical principles often unfolds through the stories of patients like Mr. John Thompson. His journey encapsulates the intricate interplay between medical facts, personal values, ethical principles, and legal considerations that healthcare professionals navigate daily.

Mr. Thompson, a 68-year-old man, finds himself in the advanced stages of a terminal illness. Despite aggressive treatment efforts, his condition has deteriorated significantly. He now endures considerable pain and discomfort, prompting the healthcare team to confront a profound ethical dilemma: should they continue with interventions that may prolong his life but also increase his suffering, or should they honor his previously expressed wishes and transition to palliative care focused on comfort?

Complicating this scenario is a divide within his family. Some members hold onto hope for a miraculous recovery, advocating for the continuation of all possible treatments. Others believe it is time to prioritize his quality of life over the extension of his lifespan. Central to this conflict is a Living Will that Mr. Thompson had thoughtfully prepared. In this advance directive, he explicitly stated his desire not to receive life-prolonging measures if there is no reasonable expectation of recovery. However, his eldest son, who holds a Durable Power of Attorney for Healthcare as his designated healthcare proxy, insists on pursuing all available treatments, believing that every possible avenue should be explored.

This situation presents a multifaceted ethical dilemma involving all four core bioethical principles: Patient Autonomy, Practitioner Beneficence, Practitioner Nonmaleficence, and Public Justice. It also brings into focus the importance of medical standards of care, decisional capacity, and the role of surrogate decision-makers.

Patient Autonomy and Informed Consent

At the heart of this case is the principle of Patient Autonomy, which underscores the right of individuals to make informed decisions about their own healthcare. Mr. Thompson's Living Will is a clear and legally binding expression of his wishes, providing specific instructions regarding his care preferences in situations where he cannot communicate them himself. This document takes precedence over surrogate decisions, legally obligating healthcare providers to honor his directives.

The healthcare team must first assess Mr. Thompson's decisional capacity. If he retains the ability to understand his condition, appreciate the consequences of treatment options, reason through the choices, and communicate his preferences, they should engage him directly in discussions about his care. However, given his advanced illness and discomfort, it is likely that he lacks this capacity, activating his advance directives.

The conflict arises with his eldest son, the designated healthcare proxy, whose insistence on continuing aggressive treatment contrasts sharply with his father's documented wishes. As an ethics consultant, you recognize the delicate balance between respecting Mr. Thompson's autonomy and addressing the emotional turmoil his son is experiencing. Your role involves facilitating open, compassionate dialogue to navigate this complex situation.

You begin by convening a meeting that includes the healthcare team and Mr. Thompson's family. Gently, you help clarify the contents and legal authority of the Living Will, ensuring that everyone understands that it reflects Mr. Thompson's own reasonable goals, values, and priorities. You acknowledge the son's love for his father and his hope for a different outcome, validating his feelings while emphasizing the ethical and legal imperatives to honor his father's expressed wishes.

Through empathetic communication, you assist the son in reconciling his desire to "do everything possible" with the reality that respecting his father's autonomy is, in fact, an act of profound love and respect. By facilitating this understanding, you help alleviate some of the moral distress he may be experiencing, guiding him toward supporting a care plan that aligns with his father's values.

Practitioner Beneficence: Maximizing Benefits

The principle of Practitioner Beneficence requires healthcare providers to act in the best interest of the patient, promoting well-being as defined by the patient's reasonable goals, values, and priorities. In Mr. Thompson's case, this means carefully considering whether continued aggressive treatment serves his best interests or merely prolongs suffering without a meaningful chance of recovery.

Transitioning to palliative care emerges as the compassionate and ethically appropriate choice. This approach focuses on alleviating pain and managing symptoms, thereby enhancing Mr. Thompson's quality of life during his remaining time. The healthcare team, guided by current medical standards of care, collaborates to develop a care plan that includes pain management specialists, social workers, and chaplaincy services. This interdisciplinary approach ensures that all aspects of Mr. Thompson's physical, emotional, and spiritual well-being are addressed.

As an ethics consultant, you support this shift by reinforcing how palliative care aligns with Mr. Thompson's expressed wishes and ethical principles. You help the family understand that this approach is not about "giving up" but about honoring his preferences and providing him with comfort and dignity.

Practitioner Nonmaleficence: Minimizing Burdens

Closely related is the principle of Practitioner Nonmaleficence, which obligates healthcare providers to avoid causing unnecessary harm or suffering. Continuing aggressive treatments in Mr. Thompson's situation may lead to increased pain, invasive procedures, and diminished quality of life without offering significant benefit.

You assist the healthcare team in evaluating the proportionality of continued interventions, weighing the potential benefits against the burdens they impose on Mr. Thompson. By focusing on pain relief and symptom management, the team actively works to minimize harm, aligning their actions with both ethical obligations and Mr. Thompson's wishes.

Your guidance helps the team and family recognize that sometimes, allowing a natural progression of illness is the most compassionate course, preventing additional suffering while providing opportunities for meaningful moments with loved ones.

Public Justice: Ensuring Fairness

The principle of Public Justice emphasizes fairness and equity within the healthcare system, ensuring that resources are used responsibly and that all patients receive equitable care. Respecting Mr. Thompson's wishes to forego further aggressive treatment aligns with this principle by avoiding the utilization of medical interventions that offer little to no benefit in his case.

You encourage transparency and fairness by facilitating open discussions about the rationale behind care decisions. This includes explaining how the proposed plan honors Mr. Thompson's values, complies with institutional policies, and aligns with societal standards of care. By doing so, you help build trust between the family and the healthcare team, reinforcing the integrity of the healthcare system.

Integrating Ethical Principles in Practice

Mr. Thompson's case serves as a summative example of how the foundational concepts of medical ethics consultation are applied in real-world scenarios. It highlights the dynamic nature of medical standards of care, the critical role of advance directives, and the complexities of surrogate decision-making.

As an ethics consultant, your multifaceted role involves:

- **Facilitating Discussions**: Navigating emotional and ethical complexities by fostering open, respectful communication among all parties.
- **Mediating Conflicts**: Helping resolve disagreements by promoting understanding and empathy.
- **Guiding Ethical Decision-Making**: Applying the four bioethical principles to ensure that care decisions are ethically sound, patient-centered, and legally compliant.

- **Educating Stakeholders**: Providing information about ethical principles, medical standards, institutional policies, and legal mandates to enhance understanding and support informed choices.
- **Ensuring Compliance**: Assisting the healthcare team in adhering to professional standards and legal requirements, including thorough documentation for accountability and transparency.

Mr. Thompson's story encapsulates the profound responsibilities and challenges inherent in medical ethics consultation. By thoughtfully applying the principles of Patient Autonomy, Practitioner Beneficence, Practitioner Nonmaleficence, and Public Justice, healthcare providers and ethics consultants can navigate complex ethical dilemmas with compassion and integrity.

This case underscores the importance of respecting patient autonomy through advance directives, the vital role of surrogate decision-makers when patients lack decisional capacity, and the necessity of aligning care decisions with medical standards of care and legal requirements. It also highlights the dynamic and context-dependent nature of these standards, emphasizing the need for continuous reflection and adaptation as medical practices evolve.

Through your involvement as an ethics consultant, you ensure that ethical considerations are not abstract concepts but integral components of patient care. You help create a healthcare environment that honors individual values, promotes well-being, minimizes harm, and upholds fairness—ultimately fostering a more compassionate and ethically aware healthcare culture.

Having explored the complexities of medical ethics in Mr. Thompson's case, it becomes evident that ethics consultants are essential in guiding patients, families, and healthcare teams through challenging decisions. We now turn to another compelling scenario that highlights the delicate balance between respecting patient autonomy and fulfilling professional responsibilities.

In the upcoming case study of Lisa—a young woman whose deeply held religious beliefs conflict with a life-saving medical intervention—we delve into the nuanced engagement required of ethics consultants. Lisa's case will further illustrate how personal convictions, cultural values, and medical ethics intersect, emphasizing the critical role of empathy, cultural sensitivity, and ethical guidance in patient care.

By examining Lisa's situation, we continue to expand our understanding of how ethical principles guide us through the most challenging scenarios, reinforcing the essential nature of thoughtful deliberation, compassion, and respect in medical ethics consultation

***

The Role of an Ethics Consultant

Ethics consultants play a multifaceted role in healthcare, providing ethical expertise, mediation, and education. They identify ethical issues, conduct comprehensive assessments, and offer recommendations that balance the four core bioethical principles: autonomy, beneficence, nonmaleficence, and justice. These recommendations must be ethically sound, legally defensible, and aligned with institutional policies and established medical standards of care.

By collaborating with interprofessional healthcare teams, ethics consultants help ensure that patient care decisions are grounded in ethical principles while complying with legal mandates and institutional guidelines. Their involvement helps foster a patient-centered approach to care, one that is ethically grounded and maintains the highest professional standards.

Case Study: Lisa

Presentation of the Case

Consider the case of Lisa, a young woman who wishes to refuse a life-saving blood transfusion due to her religious beliefs. The healthcare team is concerned about her well-being but also committed to respecting her autonomy. Lisa's case exemplifies the ethical dilemmas that arise when patient autonomy conflicts with the professional responsibility to prioritize the patient's well-being. Her decision, deeply rooted in her religious beliefs, is integral to her identity and worldview. For the healthcare team, trained to prioritize patient well-being, defining what constitutes "*well-being*" in this context is emotionally and intellectually challenging, complicating the search for a consensus.

Ethics Consultation

An ethics consultant is called in to mediate—not as a procedural formality but as a profound engagement with the values, fears, and hopes of everyone involved. You facilitate open dialogue among Lisa, her family, if Lisa permits, and the healthcare providers, ensuring that Lisa's right to autonomy is respected through informed consent. This involves carefully exploring her reasonable goals, values, and priorities, and ensuring that her decision is informed by a comprehensive understanding of the medical implications and ethical considerations.

Applying the Four Bioethical Principles

Patient Autonomy: Informed Consent

The principle of patient autonomy is crucial in the ethics consultation process, emphasizing the patient's right to make informed decisions about their care. However, this principle must be considered alongside beneficence, nonmaleficence, and public justice, as well as compliance with medical standards of care, institutional policies, and legal mandates.

In cases like Lisa's, you play a key role in ensuring that her decision is fully informed and respected. You must ensure that Lisa meets the comprehensive criteria for informed consent, which involve:

1. **Diagnosis and Prognosis:** She must comprehend her medical condition and the likely outcomes.
2. **Options:** She must be informed of all viable treatment options, including the option of no treatment.
3. **Purpose, Benefits, and Risks:** She must understand the intended outcomes of each option and be ablt to weigh the potential benefits and risks against her reasonable goals, values, and priorities.
4. **Consent:** Her consent must be made voluntarily, without any form of coercion or undue influence.

5. **Alignment:** Her consent should align with her reasonable goals, values, and priorities, and fall within the boundaries of medical standards of care, institutional policies, and legal mandates.
6. **Communication:** She must clearly express her voluntary informed consent for a treatement option, or rejection of proposed treatments.
7. **Documentation**: Practitioner must record the informed consent, or refusal of the treatment option, in the medical records.

This process involves not only explaining the medical implications of refusing a blood transfusion but also understanding how her religious convictions shape her decision.

Given the critical nature of her situation, it may be beneficial to facilitate discussions with a representative or authority figure from Lisa's religious community. This step aims to explore if there is any room for interpretation or flexibility within her beliefs that might allow for medical treatment, thereby avoiding significant harm while still respecting her faith.

Practitioner Beneficence: Maximizing Benefits

The principle of beneficence obligates healthcare providers to act in ways that promote the patient's well-being, as determined by the patient's reasonable goals, values, and priorities, focusing on what will most positively impact the patient's health and quality of life. In Lisa's case, you work with the healthcare team to explore all possible avenues that respect her autonomy while enhancing her quality of life.

This involves a careful assessment to identify treatment options that align with her reasonable goals, values, and priorities, even if they differ from standard life-saving interventions. For example, the healthcare team might consider alternative treatments that do not involve blood transfusions but still offer a chance to manage her condition effectively. By identifying such options, you help ensure that Lisa's beliefs are respected while striving to provide medical care that promotes her well-being.

Practitioner Nonmaleficence: Minimizing Burdens

The principle of nonmaleficence centers on the ethical obligation to avoid causing unnecessary harm to the patient. You play a crucial role in evaluating the potential for harm that may result from Lisa's decision to refuse a blood transfusion.

You carefully assess the risks associated with refusing the transfusion and work to balance these risks with respect for her autonomy. The goal is to find a path that minimizes harm while honoring her beliefs. This may involve exploring alternative treatments or interventions that can manage her condition without violating her religious convictions, thereby reducing the potential for harm without compromising her values.

Public Justice: Ensuring Fairness

The principle of public justice emphasizes fairness and equity in healthcare decision-making, considering the broader societal implications. You are dedicated to ensuring that all patients, including Lisa, are treated equitably and with respect for their inherent rights and dignity.

In Lisa's case, you advocate for her right to refuse treatment based on her religious beliefs while ensuring that her decision aligns with the principles of justice and fairness. You work to promote the just allocation of healthcare resources, develop policies that uphold fairness, and ensure transparent communication among all parties involved.

Comprehensive Compliance and Ethical Awareness

As an ethics consultant, you ensure that all ethical recommendations and decisions are grounded in the core bioethical principles. In cases like Lisa's, you ensure that decisions are ethically sound, legally defensible, and aligned with established medical standards of care, institutional policies, and applicable federal and state laws. Through careful consideration of patients' reasonable goals, values, and priorities, you foster a culture of ethical awareness and respect, integrating ethical decision-making into every aspect of patient care.

Broader Role in Policy Development and Ethics Education

Beyond individual cases, you contribute to the broader ethical framework within healthcare institutions. You are instrumental in developing policies that address ethical complexities, ensuring that patient care consistently reflects the core bioethical principles while complying with legal standards.

You also play a key role in ethics education, using real-world cases to train healthcare professionals. By examining cases like Lisa's in training sessions, you illustrate the practical application of ethical principles, enhancing providers' understanding of how to handle similar dilemmas. This approach encourages ongoing dialogue about ethical issues, fostering a continuous culture of ethical reflection and improvement.

Through involvement in policy development, education, and research, you ensure that ethical principles remain dynamic, evolving to meet new challenges in clinical practice. By embedding these principles into the fabric of healthcare institutions, you help build an environment where trust and transparency are paramount, and ethical principles are actively applied to enhance the quality and compassion of patient care.

Conclusion

In healthcare, ethics consultants guide complex and sensitive dilemmas, such as Lisa's case, where personal beliefs may conflict with medical recommendations. By applying the four core bioethical principles—patient autonomy, beneficence, nonmaleficence, and justice—ethics consultants ensure that patient care is ethically sound and legally defensible. Their role extends beyond individual consultations, encompassing the development of institutional policies and the education of healthcare professionals. By fostering open dialogue, promoting ethical awareness, and ensuring fairness in decision-making, ethics consultants help maintain a healthcare environment that is patient-centered, ethically grounded, and adaptable to evolving societal values.

With the growing recognition of the vital role ethics consultants play in addressing complex healthcare dilemmas, it is important to understand the roots and evolution of this essential field. The role of ethics consultants has not always been formalized, and its development reflects broader changes in medical practice, societal expectations, and advancements in healthcare technology. Tracing the historical journey of medical ethics consultation—from its origins in the Hippocratic tradition to its current professionalized form—helps illuminate the key milestones that have shaped this field and highlights the ongoing importance of ethical guidance in modern medical practice.

***

Historical Evolution of Medical Ethics Consultation

The field of medical ethics consultation has evolved significantly over time, reflecting broader changes in medical practice and societal values. Understanding this evolution enriches your perspective as an ethics consultant.

Origins in the Hippocratic Tradition

Its origins can be traced back to the Hippocratic tradition, which emphasized the moral duties of physicians. The Hippocratic Oath, regarded as the cornerstone of medical ethics, laid the groundwork for the principles of beneficence and nonmaleficence. This oath focused on the practitioner's duty to enhance patient well-being while minimizing harm, setting the stage for the development of more structured approaches to ethical decision-making in healthcare.

Emergence of Formal Ethics Consultation

Advances in Medical Technology and Patient Rights

The formal establishment of medical ethics consultation as a distinct practice began in the mid-20th century, driven by rapid advances in medical technology and a growing recognition of patient rights. Innovations such as life-support systems, organ transplants, and advanced surgical techniques introduced ethical dilemmas that extended beyond the traditional Hippocratic model. These technological advancements raised complex questions about the quality of life, definitions of death, and the equitable allocation of scarce medical resources.

Ethics consultation emerged as a necessary response to these challenges, ensuring that decisions respect patient autonomy and uphold the principles of beneficence and nonmaleficence. The need to navigate these complex ethical landscapes led to the development of more formalized ethics support within healthcare institutions.

Development of Clinical Ethics Committees

Collaborative Ethical Decision-Making

During the 1970s and 1980s, hospitals began forming clinical ethics committees, laying the groundwork for modern ethics consultation services. These committees provided platforms for addressing ethical issues collaboratively, specifying, weighing, and balancing the bioethical principles. The formation of these committees was often a response to high-profile cases and public debates about medical ethics.

The Case of Karen Ann Quinlan

One landmark case that significantly influenced the development of ethics consultation was that of Karen Ann Quinlan. In 1975, Karen, a 21-year-old woman, lapsed into a persistent vegetative state after ingesting a combination of alcohol and tranquilizers. Her parents requested the removal of her mechanical ventilator, believing it aligned with her reasonable goals, values, and priorities. The hospital initially resisted due to legal and ethical concerns about withdrawing life-sustaining treatment.

The New Jersey Supreme Court's ruling in favor of the Quinlans underscored the importance of surrogate decision-making when a patient lacks decisional capacity. The court emphasized using substituted judgment to reflect the patient's known goals, values, and priorities. When these cannot be determined, decisions should be guided by the principles of beneficence and nonmaleficence, prioritizing the patient's well-being and minimizing unnecessary suffering. This landmark decision reinforced the importance of patient autonomy through surrogate decision-making and prompted the formation of ethics committees to guide complex medical decisions involving life-sustaining treatments.

Professionalization of Ethics Consultation

Formal Training and Certification

Over time, the role of ethics consultants expanded, supported by the development of formal training programs and certification processes that professionalized the field. Professional organizations, such as the American Society for Bioethics and Humanities (ASBH), have provided frameworks for certification and ongoing education of ethics consultants. These developments have helped standardize practices, establish competencies, and promote ethical proficiency among professionals in the field.

Integral Role in Patient Care

Today, medical ethics consultation is recognized as an essential service in healthcare, contributing to the ethical and moral dimensions of patient care. Ethics consultants ensure that clinical decisions are made in accordance with ethical principles, respecting patient autonomy by considering the patient's reasonable goals, values, and priorities—even through surrogate decision-making when necessary. They promote the patient's best interests, the avoidance of harm, and the assurance of justice and fairness in patient care.

Continuing Evolution and Future Challenges

Addressing New Ethical Dilemmas

The field continues to evolve, addressing new challenges brought about by advancements in genetics, artificial intelligence, and global health disparities. For example, the rise of genetic testing and gene-editing technologies presents ethical questions about privacy, consent, and the potential for unintended consequences. Similarly, the integration of artificial intelligence in healthcare introduces concerns regarding decision-making transparency and accountability.

The Vital Role of Ethics Consultants

Ethics consultants play a vital role in ensuring that ethical considerations are integrated into every aspect of patient care, aligned with established medical standards of care, institutional policies, and legal mandates. Their work ensures that ethical principles are not just abstract ideals but are integral to everyday clinical practice. By fostering environments where patient autonomy, well-being, fairness, and compliance with ethical and legal standards are prioritized, ethics consultants help navigate the complexities of modern medicine.

Conclusion

The historical evolution of medical ethics consultation reflects the dynamic interplay between medical advancements, societal values, and ethical principles. From the foundational Hippocratic Oath to the establishment of ethics committees and professional ethics consultation services, the field has continually adapted to meet the ethical challenges of each era. High-profile cases like that of Karen Ann Quinlan have underscored the necessity of ethical guidance in complex medical decisions.

As medicine continues to advance, ethics consultants will remain essential in addressing emerging ethical dilemmas, ensuring that patient care is guided by compassion, respect, and a commitment to ethical excellence. Their role in integrating ethical considerations into clinical practice not only supports individual patient needs but also contributes to the integrity and humanity of the healthcare system as a whole.

***

Structured Ethics Consultations

For both aspiring and experienced clinical ethicists, understanding the importance of a structured approach to ethics consultations is essential to ensuring ethical clarity and consistency in patient care. Such an approach not only enhances the quality of healthcare but also ensures that ethical dilemmas are addressed systematically and thoughtfully. By providing a clear framework for deliberation, you support healthcare providers in making informed and morally sound decisions that align with the four core bioethical principles: patient autonomy, practitioner beneficence, practitioner nonmaleficence, and public justice.

Case Study: Mr. Rodriguez

Presentation of the Case

Let's delve into the case of Mr. Rodriguez, an elderly patient who has been in a persistent vegetative state for several months. He has no advance directives, and his family is divided on whether to continue life-sustaining treatment. Some family members believe that all possible measures should be taken to prolong his life, while others feel that continuing treatment only prolongs his suffering without any hope of recovery. The interprofessional healthcare team faces also an ethical dilemma: balancing the professional requirement to prioritize patient well-being—beneficence, with the requirement of avoiding harm—nonmaleficence.

Applying the Four Bioethical Principles

Patient Autonomy and Informed Consent

In situations where the patient cannot express their wishes, as with Mr. Rodriguez, the principle of patient autonomy is exercised through surrogate decision-making. Your role is to guide the legal surrogate(s) in making decisions that reflect Mr. Rodriguez's reasonable goals, values, and priorities. If these are not explicitly known, decisions should be guided by the principles of beneficence (maximizing benefits) and nonmaleficence (minimizing harm).

Structured Method for Informed Consent:

1. **Diagnosis and Prognosis:** Ensure that the legal surrogate(s) receive detailed and understandable information about Mr. Rodriguez's medical condition, prognosis, and the implications of continuing or withdrawing life-sustaining treatment.
2. **Treatment Options:** Discuss all available options, including the continuation of current treatment, the introduction of new interventions, or the withdrawal of life support in favor of palliative care.
3. **Purposes:** Clearly explain the intended purpose of each option, whether it is to prolong life, alleviate suffering, or provide comfort.
4. **Benefits and Risks:** Help the surrogate(s) assess the potential benefits and burdens associated with each option, considering Mr. Rodriguez's quality of life.
5. **Consent:** Ensure that the legal surrogate(s) provide informed consent, supported by logical reasoning that aligns with Mr. Rodriguez's reasonable goals, values, and priorities. If these are unknown, decisions should be guided by the principles of beneficence (maximizing benefits) and nonmaleficence (minimizing harm). Either way, they must in compliance with institutional policies, legal requirements, and medical standards of care.
6. **Documentation**: The surrogate(s) informed consent must be communicated clearly and documented in the medical records.

By following this structured method, you help ensure that the necessary conditions for informed consent are met, even when the patient cannot participate directly. This respects patient autonomy by proxy and provides consistency in the decision-making process.

It also ensures compliance with ethical principles, medical standards of care, legal requirements, institutional policies, and clear documentation for accountability and transparency.

Practitioner Beneficence: Maximizing Benefits

The principle of beneficence requires acting in the patient's best interest to promote their well-being. In Mr. Rodriguez's case, this involves carefully evaluating whether continued life-sustaining treatment serves his best interests or merely prolongs suffering.

Structured Approach to Beneficence:

Systematic Evaluation: Collaborate with the interprofessional healthcare team to systematically consider and evaluate all treatment options that:

- align with Mr. Rodriguez's reasonable goals, values, and priorities,
- adhere to established medical standards of care,
- comply with institutional policies, and
- fulfill all applicable legal requirements.

By adhering to this structured approach, you help the healthcare team focus on promoting Mr. Rodriguez's well-being in a manner consistent with ethical principles and legal requirements. This systematic process fosters consistency and reliability in ethical decision-making.

Practitioner Nonmaleficence: Minimizing Burdens

Nonmaleficence obligates healthcare providers to avoid causing unnecessary harm. Continuing life-sustaining treatment for Mr. Rodriguez might lead to prolonged suffering without the prospect of recovery.

Structured Ethical Analysis for Nonmaleficence:

Identifying Potential Harms: Systematically assess the physical, emotional, and psychological harms associated with each treatment option. This process involves carefully weighing and balancing the potential benefits of each option against the risks and burdens they may impose on Mr. Rodriguez. These considerations should be guided by:

- Mr. Rodriguez's reasonable goals, values, and priorities,
- established medical standards of care,
- relevant institutional policies, and
- applicable legal mandates and prohibitions.

By conducting this analysis, you provide clarity in navigating complex ethical dilemmas, ensuring that actions are guided by thorough ethical consideration that prioritizes patient safety and well-being.

Public Justice: Ensuring Fairness

Public justice requires that healthcare decisions are made with fairness and equity, considering the broader societal implications.

Structured Method for Public Justice:

- **Transparent Decision-Making**: Facilitate open, honest discussions that include all relevant stakeholders, such as the legal surrogate(s) and the interprofessional healthcare team.
- **Consistent Criteria**: Ensure that decisions are guided by consistent ethical principles, avoiding any form of bias or favoritism.
- **Fair Allocation of Resources**: Advocate for the equitable allocation of healthcare resources, ensuring that Mr. Rodriguez receives care that is fair and just.

Using this structured approach, you help ensure that all patients are treated fairly, and decisions are aligned with societal expectations and ethical principles. This fosters trust and integrity within the healthcare system.

Comprehensive Compliance and Ethical Awareness

In the complex landscape of healthcare, your role is critical in ensuring that all ethical recommendations and decisions are firmly grounded in the core bioethical principles. By adhering to a structured process, you foster a culture of ethical awareness and respect that permeates all aspects of patient care. This approach supports healthcare professionals in consistently making ethical decisions that uphold the dignity and rights of patients.

Broader Role in Policy Development and Ethics Education

Beyond individual cases, you contribute to the broader ethical framework within healthcare institutions. Drawing from cases like Mr. Rodriguez's, you can:

- **Policy Development:** Help create policies that guide ethical decision-making in complex cases, ensuring consistency and fairness.
- **Ethics Education:** Use real-world cases to train healthcare professionals, enhancing their understanding of ethical principles and improving their ability to navigate ethical dilemmas.
- **Research Advancement:** Participate in research to inform best practices and advance the field of medical ethics.

By embedding ethical principles into policy development, education, and research, you ensure that decisions are made with a full appreciation of their ethical implications.

Conclusion

Structured ethics consultations are essential tools for navigating the complex ethical dilemmas that arise in healthcare. Through the systematic application of the four core bioethical principles, you guide healthcare teams in making decisions that respect patient autonomy, promote well-being, minimize harm, and ensure fairness. Cases like Mr. Rodriguez's demonstrate that ethical consultation is not merely about theoretical ideals but about practical, patient-centered solutions that uphold the dignity and rights of every individual.

By providing a structured framework for ethical decision-making, you enhance the integrity and compassion of patient care. Your work plays a vital role in policy development and ethics education, ensuring that ethical principles remain dynamic and responsive to new challenges in clinical practice. This fosters a culture of ethical awareness and accountability, integral to the mission of healthcare institutions committed to excellence in patient care.

***

The Bioethics Program

Mission Statement

The mission of the Bioethics Program is to provide ethics consultation, education, and policy development grounded in the four core bioethical principles:

Patient Autonomy (Informed Consent): Respecting the patient's right to make informed decisions about their treatment options. This requires the following steps:

- **Diagnosis and Prognosis:** Patients or their legal surrogates must fully understand the medical condition and its likely progression.
- **Options:** They must be informed of all viable treatment options, including the option to decline treatment.
- **Benefits and Risks:** Patients or their surrogates must comprehend the potential outcomes of each option, weighing the benefits and risks in alignment with the patient's reasonable goals, values, and priorities.
- **Informed Consent:** Consent must be given voluntarily, free from coercion, and with a full understanding of the decisions being made. The process of informed consent should be revisited as the patient's condition or available treatment options change.
- **Alignment:** Decisions must align with the patient's reasonable goals, values, and priorities, while also meeting medical standards of care, institutional policies, and legal requirements.
- **Documentation:** The patient's informed consent must be clearly communicated and properly documented in the medical records.

Practitioner Beneficence (Maximizing Benefits): Acting in the best interest of the patient to promote their well-being, guided by the patient's reasonable goals, values, and priorities. All actions must comply with medical standards of care, institutional policies, and legal requirements. Practitioners should work collaboratively with the interprofessional healthcare team to ensure the best possible outcomes while balancing innovative treatments that remain within the boundaries of established medical standards.

Practitioner Nonmaleficence (Minimizing Burdens): Avoiding treatment options that cause unnecessary harm or suffering to the patient. The goal is to minimize harm by considering the patient's reasonable goals, values, and priorities, ensuring that all actions conform to medical standards of care, institutional policies, and legal requirements. Practitioners must carefully balance the principles of beneficence and nonmaleficence, recognizing that treatments intended to benefit the patient may also carry risks of harm. The goal is to minimize harm while promoting the patient's overall well-being, even when facing complex medical decisions.

Public Justice (Ensuring Fairness): Ensuring that all patients receive equitable and fair treatment within the healthcare system. This involves adherence to institutional, state, and federal laws, as well as ethical and professional standards, ensuring that care and resources are distributed ethically without bias or favoritism. Public justice also entails addressing systemic healthcare disparities—such as those based on race, socioeconomic status, and geographic location—by promoting equitable access to care for all patients, especially vulnerable populations. The program is committed to identifying and mitigating these disparities to ensure fair treatment and the equitable distribution of healthcare resources.

The Bioethics Program is committed to fostering ethical awareness, continuous education, and leadership in ethical decision-making, ensuring that ethical considerations are integrated into all aspects of patient care and organizational policy.

Key Elements

- **Purpose and Objectives:** To provide ethics consultation, education, and policy development that support and enhance ethical decision-making across the healthcare system.
- **Ethical Foundation:** Ensuring that all actions taken within the program are grounded in the core bioethical principles—autonomy, beneficence, nonmaleficence, and public justice—which guide every aspect of patient care and policy development.
- **Practitioner's Role:** Outlining the professional responsibility of practitioners to ensure that patients fully comprehend their diagnosis, available treatment options, and associated benefits and risks. Practitioners must help patients make informed decisions that align with their reasonable goals, values, and priorities, while adhering to medical standards of care, institutional policies, and legal requirements. Practitioners are not only responsible for ensuring these decisions are documented but also for actively guiding patients through the ethical decision-making process.
- **Patient's Role:** Patients, or their surrogates, have the right to fully understand their diagnosis, treatment options, and risks, enabling them to make informed decisions that align with their personal goals, values, and priorities, within the boundaries of medical standards of care, institutional policies, and legal requirements.
- **Leadership in Ethics:** Highlighting the program's responsibility in fostering ethical awareness and providing leadership in ethical decision-making. This includes developing policies, facilitating ethics consultations, and educating healthcare professionals about ethical principles in practice.

Vision Statement

The vision of the Bioethics Program is to create a healthcare environment where ethical principles are central to all clinical and organizational decisions. By fostering a healthcare environment rooted in ethical reflection, dialogue, and education, the program ensures that ethical leadership permeates both clinical practice and organizational decision-making.

The Bioethics Program will provide leadership and oversight in ethics consultation and policy development, ensuring that ethical principles are not only applied to patient care but also shape broader organizational policies and healthcare standards. Patient choices will be respected within the boundaries of ethically appropriate treatment options, thereby enhancing the quality, integrity, and compassion of care.

Key Elements

- **Long-Term Goals:** Envisioning a future where all decisions are guided by the balanced consideration of ethical principles, thoughtfully integrating autonomy, beneficence, nonmaleficence, and justice.
- **Ethical Culture:** Promoting a culture of continuous ethical reflection, dialogue, and collaboration among all healthcare practitioners.
- **Integration of Principles:** Underscoring the importance of specifying, weighing, and balancing bioethical principles within medical standards of care, institutional policies, and legal mandates.
- **Leadership and Oversight:** Emphasizing the program's commitment to providing leadership in ethics consultation and policy development, shaping both patient care and organizational behavior.

Values Statement

The values of the Bioethics Program are grounded in the principles of patient autonomy, practitioner beneficence, practitioner nonmaleficence, and public justice. These principles guide every action taken by the program, ensuring that patient care, policy development, and organizational practices are consistently aligned with established ethical standards, medical standards of care, institutional policies, and legal mandates.

The program is committed to embedding these values into all aspects of patient care and decision-making, providing leadership in ethical practice, and fostering an environment where ethical considerations are a fundamental part of both clinical practice and organizational behavior.

Key Elements

- **Core Bioethical Principles:** Emphasizing the foundational principles of patient autonomy, practitioner beneficence, practitioner nonmaleficence, and public justice that guide the Bioethics Program.
- **Alignment with Standards:** Ensuring that all actions are consistently aligned with ethical standards, medical standards of care, institutional policies, and legal mandates.
- **Integration into Practice:** Embedding these values into patient care, policy development, and organizational behavior to ensure that ethical considerations are a fundamental part of decision-making processes.
- **Commitment to Ethical Leadership:** Fostering leadership in ethical practice by promoting an environment where ethical awareness is actively supported and integrated into both clinical practice and organizational conduct.

***

The Tripartite Process

TAC Methodology in Ethics Consultation

Building upon the mission, vision, and values statements, effective ethics consultation in healthcare requires a deliberate and systematic approach to navigating complex ethical dilemmas. The **Tripartite Process—Think, Assess, and Conclude (TAC)**—provides a structured framework that guides practitioners and ethics consultants through the intricate terrain of ethical decision-making. This framework ensures that all considerations are thoroughly examined before arriving at a resolution, upholding the highest standards of ethical integrity and compliance with institutional policies and legal mandates.

Foundation of the TAC Methodology

While the TAC methodology is firmly grounded in the four core bioethical principles, the selection of these specific principles is rooted in the historical and philosophical traditions of medical ethics. Originating from the Hippocratic Oath, these principles have evolved to address the broader ethical challenges faced in modern healthcare. Their long-standing tradition, philosophical coherence, and practical applicability have led to their adoption as part of the medical standard of care, institutional policies, and legal requirments, forming the foundation of the TAC methodology.

Think: Identifying the Ethical Issue

The first step is to **Think**—a careful and deliberate determination of the ethical issue at hand. This involves:

- **Reflective Analysis:** Engaging in introspection to understand the core ethical concern.
- **Challenging Assumptions:** Questioning preconceived notions to uncover underlying issues.

- **Defining the Problem:** Clearly articulating the ethical dilemma to lay the groundwork for further analysis.

This step is critical as it ensures that subsequent actions are appropriately targeted and ethically sound.

Assess: Specifying, Weighing, and Balancing the Four Principles

The next step is to **Assess** the situation by specifying, weighing, and balancing the four core principles:

1. **Patient Autonomy** (Informed Consent)
2. **Practitioner Beneficence** (Maximizing Benefits)
3. **Practitioner Nonmaleficence** (Minimizing Burdens)
4. **Public Justice** (Ensuring Fairness)

During this phase:

- **Principlism Application:** Analyze how each principle applies to the specific circumstances.
- **Evaluate Importance:** Assess the relative importance of each principle in the context.
- **Balance Principles:** Align them with the patient's reasonable goals, values, and priorities.

This ensures that the patient's best interests are maximized within the framework of medical standards of care, institutional policies, and legal mandates.

Conclude: Reaching an Ethical Resolution

The final step is to **Conclude** by determining an ethically appropriate resolution that is consistent with established medical standards of care, institutional policies, and legal mandates. This involves:

- **Contextual Resolution:** Arriving at a solution that addresses the specific ethical issues identified.

- **Alignment with Standards:** Ensuring the consent is in accordance with medical standards of care, institutional policies, and legal requirements.
- **Implementation:** Outlining actionable steps to put the ethical resolution into practice.

This structured approach ensures that decisions are well-considered, ethically justifiable, and practically implementable.

Core Ethical Principles in Practice

Patient Autonomy: Informed Consent

At the heart of patient autonomy is the fundamental right of patients to make informed decisions about their healthcare. This involves:

1. **Diagnosis and Prognosis:** Patients, or their surrogate(s), must comprehend their medical condition and the likely course it will take.
2. **Available Options:** Being informed of all viable treatment options, including the option of no treatment.
3. **Purpose, Benefits, and Risks:** Understanding the intended outcomes of each option and weighing the potential benefits and risks against their reasonable goals, values, and priorities.
4. **Consent:** Ensuring that medical decisions are made voluntarily, without any form of coercion.
5. **Alignment:** Consent should align with the patient's reasonable goals, values, and priorities, and fall within the boundaries of medical standards of care, institutional policies, and legal mandates.
6. **Documentation:** Clearly expressing informed consent or informed rejection of proposed treatments and documenting it in the medical records.

Role of Surrogates

When a patient lacks decisional capacity, a legally established surrogate(s) uses substituted judgment to reflect the patient's reasonable goals, values, and priorities. If these are unknown, decisions are guided by nonmaleficence and beneficence to prioritize the patient's well-being.

Practitioner Responsibility: Upholding Professional Integrity

Practitioners have a dual obligation to respect patient autonomy while adhering to ethical, professional, and legal standards. This involves:

- **Presenting Evidence-Based Options:** Offering treatment options that are scientifically validated and pose minimal risk.
- **Effective Communication:** Conveying complex medical information in understandable terms.
- **Ethical Practice:** Upholding the principles of beneficence and nonmaleficence to promote patient well-being and avoid harm.

Public Policy: The Foundation of Ethical Standards

Public policy establishes ethical standards for medical practice, ensuring:

- **Equitable Care:** Delivering healthcare services without discrimination.
- **Resource Allocation:** Fair distribution of resources to minimize disparities.
- **Advocacy:** Engaging in policy development to uphold justice and fairness, especially during public health crises.

Integrating TAC with SOAP: Documenting Ethical Analysis

To ensure effective communication and integration into the clinical workflow, the TAC methodology can be documented using the **SOAP** (**S**ubjective, **O**bjective, **A**ssessment, **P**lan) format.

1. **S** (Subjective): Capture the patient's perspective, including their understanding of their condition, their goals, values, and priorities, as well as any ethical concerns they may have.
2. **O** (Objective): Record observable data such as medical history, current condition, applicable policies, laws, and ethical principles involved.
3. **A** (Assessment): Document the TAC methodology to analyze the situation, specifying, weighing, and balancing the ethical principles to reach a conclusion.
4. **P** (Plan): Outline the proposed course of action, including recommendations and steps to align with medical standards and legal mandates.

This combined approach ensures that ethical analysis is clearly communicated, actionable, and integrated into the patient's care plan.

Conclusion

The **Think, Assess, Conclude (TAC)** methodology offers a structured approach to ethics consultation, ensuring that ethical dilemmas are addressed with rigor, compassion, and integrity. By balancing patient autonomy with practitioner responsibilities and public policy requirements, this approach helps ensure decisions are ethically sound and aligned with the highest standards of medical care and legal mandates.

Incorporating the SOAP format strengthens the ethical foundations of clinical decision-making, ensuring decisions are clearly documented and consistent with professional and legal standards. Through this integration, healthcare professionals are equipped with a common moral language, enabling them to navigate the complex landscape of modern healthcare ethics effectively.

As you continue your journey as an aspiring or experienced clinical ethicist, remember that each case you encounter is an opportunity to apply these principles and methodologies. Your role is not only to resolve ethical dilemmas but also to foster an environment where ethical considerations are integral to healthcare. By doing so, you enhance the quality and compassion of patient care, contributing to a more ethical and just healthcare system.

***

The following templates and checklists are designed to ensure that the interprofessional healthcare teams, including the ethics consultants, have the necessary tools to conduct thorough, ethical, and well-documented consultations and policy developments. They will help in maintaining consistency, transparency, completeness, and accountability.

***

1.1 Ethics Consultation Intake Form

Purpose: To gather all necessary information at the start of an ethics consultation, ensuring that the consultant has a complete understanding of the situation.

Patient Name: ______________________________
Date of Birth: ______________________________
Medical Record Number: ______________________
Primary Diagnosis: __________________________
Current Treatment Plan: ______________________

Consultation Requestor
Name: ______________________________________
Role/Title: __________________________________
Department: _________________________________
Contact Information: __________________________

Reason for Consultation

- **Primary Ethical Issue(s)**: [Brief description of the ethical issue(s) prompting the consultation]
- **Specific Questions for the Ethics Consultant**: [List any specific questions or concerns that need to be addressed]

Involved Parties

- ☐ **Patient**:
- ☐ **Family Members**: [List names if applicable]
- ☐ **Healthcare Team Members**: [List names and roles]
- ☐ **Others**: (e.g., legal, social work, clergy): [List names and roles]

Urgency of the Consultation —

- ☐ **Immediate** (within hours)
- ☐ **Soon** (within 24-48 hours)
- ☐ **Routine** (within a few days)

Preliminary Information Gathered

- **Advance Directives**:
  - ☐ Yes
  - ☐ No

  [Brief description if applicable]
- **Capacity Assessment**:
  - ☐ Yes
  - ☐ No

  [Details if applicable]
- **Family Dynamics**:

  [Brief description if relevant]
- **Cultural/Religious Considerations**:
  - ☐ Yes
  - ☐ No

  [Brief description if applicable]

Initial Ethical Analysis by Requestor

- [Brief summary of any ethical considerations identified by the requestor]

Date/Time of Request: ______________________________

Consultant Assigned: ______________________________

***

1.2 TAC Methodology & SOAP Documentation

Purpose: To provide a structured framework for ethical consultation and decision-making, focusing on the bioethical principles of Patient Autonomy, Practitioner Beneficence, Practitioner Nonmaleficence, and Public Justice.

Patient Name: ______________________________
Date of Birth: ______________________________
Medical Record Number: ______________________
Primary Diagnosis: __________________________
Current Treatment Plan: ______________________

(T) THINK

- **Ethical Dilemma**: Articulate the ethical dilemma or topic clearly.
- **Case Details**: Gather and review case details, including medical history and patient circumstances.
- **Boundaries**: Ensure a thorough understanding of medical standards of care, institutional policies, and legal mandates and prohibitions.
- **Stakeholders**: Identify all individuals and entities impacted by the ethical issue (e.g., patient, family, healthcare team, institution, community). Consider broader impacts, such as societal or public health implications, if relevant.

(A) ASSESS

1. **Patient Autonomy** (Informed Consent):
   - **Specification**: The practitioner has determined that the patient or surrogate has provided informed consent.
   - **Informed Consent's Necessary Conditions:**
     (all boxes must be checked for informed consent)
     - ☐ **Decisional Capacity**: The patient or surrogate has the ability to understand and make informed decisions about their care.
     - ☐ **Diagnosis and Prognosis**: They comprehend their medical condition and the likely outcomes.
     - ☐ **Options**: All viable treatment options, including the option of no treatment, have been presented.
     - ☐ **Purposes, Benefits, and Risks**: They understand the intended outcomes of each option and can weigh the potential benefits and risks against their reasonable goals, values, and priorities.
     - ☐ **Consent**: The consent is voluntary, free from pressure or coercion; practitioners should assess and document any signs or sources of coercion.
     - ☐ **Alignment**: The treatment decision aligns with the patient's reasonable goals, values, and priorities and falls within the boundaries of medical standards of care, institutional policies, and legal mandates.
     - ☐ **Documentation**: The patient's or surrogate's informed consent has been clearly communicated to the appropriate individuals, documented in the medical records, and shared with all relevant healthcare team members.

2. **Practitioner Beneficence** (Maximize Benefits):

- **Specification**: Practitioner has determined that beneficence is being implemented with the treatment options that will be presented to the patient.
- **Beneficence's Necessary Conditions:**
  (all boxes must be checked for compliance)
  - ☐ **Maximization**: The practitioner's treatment options maximize the patient's best interests, as determined by the patient's reasonable goals, values, and priorities.
  - ☐ **Boundaries**: The practitioner's treatment options comply with medical standards of care, institutional policies, and legal mandates and prohibitions.
  - ☐ **Review**: Decisions to maximize benefits should be revisited regularly as patient conditions and circumstances change.

---

3. **Practitioner Nonmaleficence** (Minimize Burdens):

- **Specification**: Practitioner has determined that nonmaleficence is being implemented with the treatment options that will be presented to the patient.
- **Nonmaleficence's Necessary Conditions:**
  (all boxes must be checked for compliance)
  - ☐ **Minimization**: The practitioner's treatment options minimize the patient's burdens, as determined by the patient's reasonable goals, values, and priorities.
  - ☐ **Boundaries**: The practitioner's treatment options comply with medical standards of care, institutional policies, and legal mandates and prohibitions.

4. **Public Justice** (Ensure Fairness):

- **Specification**: Practitioner determines that justice as fairness is being implemented.
- **Justice's Necessary Conditions:**
  (all boxes must be checked for compliance)
  - ☐ **Fairness**: The practitioner's treatment options promote fairness.
  - ☐ **Boundaries**: The practitioner's treatment options comply with medical standards of care, institutional policies, and legal mandates and prohibitions.

(C) CONCLUDE

- ☐ **Weigh**: The patient/surrogate and practitioner must jointly determine the relative weights of each of the four specified principles, considering the patient's reasonable goals, values, and priorities, medical standards of care, institutional policies, and legal mandates and prohibitions.
- ☐ **Balance**: The patient/surrogate and practitioner must jointly determine which principle, or groups of principles, guide the decision-making towards a rational and reasonable recommendation or decision.
- ☐ **Communicate**: Clearly document and communicate the agreed-upon decision to all relevant parties to ensure understanding and alignment.

DOCUMENTATION:

SOAP Notes:

- ☐ **(S) Subjective**: Document the patient's or surrogate's perspective on the medical condition, diagnosis, prognosis, and treatment options, including their ethical considerations.
- ☐ **(O) Objective**: Record objective medical facts, such as diagnosis, clinical observations, and test results. Ensure all facts align with current medical standards of care.
- ☐ **(A) Assessment**: Evaluate the ethical issues identified, summarizing the THINK and ASSESS steps, and document the TAC analysis with reference to each bioethical principle.
- ☐ **(P) Plan**: Develop a plan that outlines the recommended course of action, including steps for communicating findings and recommendations to all stakeholders. Document how the decision adheres to ethical principles, medical standards of care, and legal requirements.

Consultant Name: ______________________________

Date: ___________

***

1.3 Ethics Consultation Debrief Checklist

Purpose: To guide a structured debriefing session after an ethics consultation, helping the team reflect on the process, decisions made, and areas for improvement.

Patient Name: ______________________________
Consultation Date: ___________________________
Primary Ethical Issue(s): [Brief summary]

Debrief Participants

- [List names and roles of participants in the debriefing session]

Effectiveness of the Consultation Process

- ☐ Process was clear and well-organized
- ☐ All relevant parties were included and heard

Ethical Analysis and Decision-Making

- ☐ The principles of bioethics were appropriately applied
- ☐ Cultural, religious, and social factors were adequately considered

Communication and Interaction

- ☐ Communication was clear and respectful among all parties
- ☐ All misunderstandings and conflicts were addressed

Outcome and Follow-Up

- ☐ Outcome aligned with the patient's reasonable goals, values, and priorities
- ☐ Outcome is compliant with medical standards of care, institutional policies, and legal mandates and prohibitions
- ☐ Follow-up actions have been addressed

Lessons Learned

- What worked well in this consultation?
- What could be improved for future consultations?

Emotional Impact

- How did the consultation affect the participants emotionally?
- Are any additional support or resources needed?

Next Steps

- **Action Items**: [List any actions to be taken based on the debriefing session]
- **Follow-Up Consultation**:
  ☐ Yes [If Yes, specify timing and purpose]
  ☐ No
- **Documentation**: [Ensure all documentation is complete and accurate]

Debrief Leader Name: ______________________________
Date/Time Completed: ______________________________

***

1.4 Policy Development Template

Purpose: To provide a structured and comprehensive framework for developing, implementing, and maintaining clear, legally compliant, and ethically robust policies within the organization.

Policy Title: [Title of the Policy]
Policy Number: [Assign a unique policy number]
Date of Creation/Revision: [Date the policy was created or last revised]
Effective Date:[Date the policy comes into effect]
Review Date: [Scheduled date for the policy review]

Purpose

- Clearly state the purpose of the policy, including its objectives, the issues it addresses, and what it aims to achieve within the organization.

Scope

- Define the scope of the policy, including:
  - The individuals, departments, or processes to which the policy applies.
  - Any specific circumstances or contexts under which the policy is applicable.

Definitions

- Provide clear definitions for any key terms used within the policy to ensure understanding and consistency in interpretation.

Policy Statement

- Articulate the core principles, ethical standards, and key guidelines upon which the policy is based. This section should be a concise declaration of the policy's intentions and overarching framework.

Procedures

- Detail the specific steps required to implement and comply with the policy. This should include:
  - **Step-by-Step Guidelines:** A detailed description of the procedures to be followed.
  - **Documentation Requirements:** Outline any forms, checklists, or documentation that must be completed as part of the process.

Responsibilities

- Clearly assign and describe the roles and responsibilities of individuals or departments involved in the implementation and oversight of the policy.

Legal, Ethical, and Compliance Considerations

- Identify and discuss any relevant laws, regulations, ethical guidelines, or institutional standards that the policy must adhere to. Ensure that the policy aligns with both legal and ethical requirements.

Training and Education

- Describe any training or educational initiatives required to effectively implement the policy. Specify the target audience, training content, and delivery methods.

Monitoring, Compliance, and Evaluation

- Outline the mechanisms for monitoring adherence to the policy, including:
  - **Compliance Monitoring:** Methods for ensuring that the policy is followed, such as audits or reporting requirements.
  - **Evaluation:** Processes for assessing the effectiveness of the policy and its impact.
  - **Enforcement:** Describe any enforcement actions or consequences for non-compliance.

Review and Revision Process

- Detail the process for reviewing and revising the policy, including:

- **Frequency of Review:** How often the policy should be reviewed.
- **Process for Revision:** Steps for making revisions, including who is responsible for the review and how revisions will be approved.

Related Policies and Documents

- List any related policies, procedures, or documents that should be consulted in conjunction with this policy to ensure comprehensive coverage of the subject matter.

Approval

- Include a section for formal approval, noting the authorities responsible for finalizing and approving the policy.

Approved by: [Name and Title]
Date of Approval: [Approval Date]

Appendices

- Attach or reference any supplementary documents, forms, or additional materials that support the policy.

***

Review Questions

True/False Questions:

1. Medical ethics consultation is primarily designed to resolve medical errors rather than address ethical dilemmas.
True or False?

2. Ethics consultants help ensure that patient care decisions are made with consideration of ethical principles.
True or False?

3. The role of ethics consultants includes policy development and ethics education.
True or False?

4. The principle of beneficence in bioethics emphasizes doing no harm to the patient.
True or False?

5. The establishment of clinical ethics committees began in the mid-20th century.
True or False?

Multiple-Choice Questions:

6. Which of the following best describes the primary aim of medical ethics consultation?
a) To enforce legal standards in healthcare
b) To reduce healthcare costs
c) To enhance the quality of patient care by integrating ethical considerations
d) To provide medical treatment options

7. What is the principle of nonmaleficence in bioethics?
a) Acting in the patient's best interest
b) Ensuring fairness in healthcare
c) Respecting patient choices and autonomy
d) Avoiding harm to the patient

Clinical Vignettes:

8. **Scenario:** Mr. Rodriguez, an elderly patient in a persistent vegetative state with no advance directives, has a family divided on whether to continue life-sustaining treatment. The healthcare team is unsure how to proceed. What is the best course of action?
a) Continue life-sustaining treatment indefinitely
b) Withdraw life-sustaining treatment immediately
c) Involve an ethics consultant to facilitate discussions and reach a consensus
d) Make a decision based on the healthcare team's majority opinion

9. **Scenario:** Lisa, a young woman, refuses a life-saving blood transfusion due to her religious beliefs. The interprofessional healthcare team is concerned about her well-being but also wants to respect her autonomy. What is the best course of action?
a) Force the blood transfusion to save her life
b) Respect her decision without further discussion
c) Call an ethics consultant to mediate and explore a respectful solution
d) Transfer her to another hospital

10. **Scenario:** Mrs. Patel decides to refuse a recommended surgery despite understanding the potential consequences. The interprofessional healthcare team is unsure if her decision is truly informed. What is the best course of action?
a) Proceed with the surgery against her wishes
b) Respect her decision without verifying
c) Ensure a thorough informed consent process to confirm her decision is informed
d) Involve her family to make the decision on her behalf

Correct Answers:

1. False (Medical ethics consultation is primarily designed to address ethical dilemmas in patient care, not just to resolve medical errors. It involves guiding patients, families, and healthcare providers through complex ethical issues to ensure decisions are made in alignment with ethical principles.)
2. True
3. True
4. False (The principle of beneficence in bioethics emphasizes doing good and promoting the well-being of the patient. The principle of nonmaleficence is the one that specifically emphasizes doing no harm.)
5. True
6. c) To enhance the quality of patient care by integrating ethical considerations
7. d) Avoiding harm to the patient
8. c) Involve an ethics consultant to facilitate discussions and reach a consensus
9. c) Call an ethics consultant to mediate and explore a respectful solution
10. c) Ensure a thorough informed consent process to confirm her decision is informed

***

Further Readings and References

- Beauchamp, T. L., & Childress, J. F. (2019). Principles of Biomedical Ethics (8th ed.). Oxford University Press.
  - *This foundational text provides an in-depth discussion of the four principles of biomedical ethics: autonomy, beneficence, nonmaleficence, and justice.*
- Jonsen, A. R., Siegler, M., & Winslade, W. J. (2015). Clinical Ethics: A Practical Approach to Ethical Decisions in Clinical Medicine (8th ed.). McGraw-Hill Education.
  - *A practical guide to addressing ethical dilemmas in clinical practice, with case studies and frameworks for decision-making.*
- American Society for Bioethics and Humanities (ASBH). (2011). Core Competencies for Healthcare Ethics Consultation. ASBH.
  - *This document outlines the essential skills and knowledge required for healthcare ethics consultants, emphasizing the role of ethics consultation in clinical practice.*
- Quill, T. E., & Cassel, C. K. (1995). "*Nonabandonment: A Central Obligation for Physicians.*" Annals of Internal Medicine, 122(5), 368-374.
  - *An article discussing the ethical obligation of nonabandonment in the physician-patient relationship, relevant to the role of ethics consultants in ensuring continuous care.*
- Fins, J. J., & Bacchetta, M. D. (1995). "*Framing the Clinical Ethics Case Consultation: A Pedagogical and Problem-Oriented Approach.*" Journal of Clinical Ethics, 6(3), 239-251.
  - *This article offers a pedagogical approach to conducting ethics consultations, focusing on case framing and problem-solving strategies.*

- Aulisio, M. P., Arnold, R. M., & Youngner, S. J. (2000). "*Health Care Ethics Consultation: Nature, Goals, and Competencies.*" In J. Sugarman & D. P. Sulmasy (Eds.), Methods in Medical Ethics (pp. 180-196). Georgetown University Press.
  - *A comprehensive overview of the nature and goals of healthcare ethics consultation, along with the competencies required for effective practice.*
- Pellegrino, E. D., & Thomasma, D. C. (1993). The Virtues in Medical Practice. Oxford University Press.
  - *A philosophical exploration of the virtues essential to medical practice, including the role of ethics consultation in promoting virtuous behavior in healthcare.*
- Truog, R. D., Campbell, M. L., Curtis, J. R., Haas, C. E., Luce, J. M., Rubenfeld, G. D., Rushton, C. H., & Kaufman, D. C. (2008). "*Recommendations for End-of-Life Care in the Intensive Care Unit: A Consensus Statement by the American College of Critical Care Medicine.*" Critical Care Medicine, 36(3), 953-963.
  - *Consensus recommendations on end-of-life care in the ICU, highlighting the ethical considerations and the role of ethics consultation in decision-making.*
- Zoloth, L. (2002). Health Care and the Ethics of Encounter: A Jewish Discussion of Social Justice. University of North Carolina Press.
  - *A discussion of social justice in healthcare from a Jewish ethical perspective, relevant to the principle of justice in bioethics.*
- Post, S. G., Blustein, J., Gordon, E. J., & Mishkin, D. (Eds.). (2007). Handbook for Health Care Ethics Committees. Johns Hopkins University Press.
  - *A practical guide for ethics committees, with chapters on conducting ethics consultations, policy development, and ethics education.*

***

Part II: The Ethics Consultation Process

Initiating an Ethics Consultation

Ethics consultations are a critical component in managing complex ethical dilemmas in healthcare. They provide a structured and systematic approach to addressing ethical conflicts that arise when there are tensions between patient preferences, medical recommendations, institutional policies, or legal requirements. These consultations ensure that ethical considerations are fully integrated into patient care, aligning with the Bioethics Program's mission and vision statements.

Identifying the Need for Consultation

An ethics consultation is typically required in situations where there is a conflict between a patient's or surrogate's wishes and the recommendations of the healthcare team, uncertainties regarding the ethically appropriate course of action, or disputes among family members and healthcare providers about the patient's care. Identifying the need for an ethics consultation is the first step in resolving these issues.

Healthcare practitioners, patients, or family members may identify situations that call for ethical guidance, especially when they involve critical decisions that impact the patient's quality of life, autonomy, or when there is ambiguity in interpreting the patient's reasonable goals, values, and priorities. Recognizing these needs early ensures that ethical issues are addressed proactively, minimizing the risk of prolonged conflict and distress.

Requesting and Referring Ethics Consultations

The process of requesting an ethics consultation should be streamlined and clearly defined to ensure that requests are handled promptly and efficiently. Establishing clear protocols is essential. These protocols should outline:

- **Criteria for Initiating a Consultation**: The criteria should include situations where patient autonomy is in question, where the potential benefits and harms of treatment options need careful weighing, or where justice concerns arise due to the allocation of resources.
- **Process for Submitting a Request**: A standardized process for submitting requests ensures consistency. Requests can come from any member of the healthcare team, patients, or family members. They should be made through a designated channel, such as an ethics consultation request form or direct referral to the ethics committee.
- **Roles and Responsibilities**: Defining the roles and responsibilities of those involved in the consultation process helps maintain clarity and accountability. The roles may include the ethics consultant, healthcare practitioners, patients, surrogates, and other relevant stakeholders.

Setting Goals and Objectives for Ethics Consultations

Once an ethics consultation is initiated, it is imperative to establish clear goals and objectives to guide the process. This involves identifying the specific ethical issues at hand, defining the desired outcomes, and outlining the necessary steps to achieve these outcomes. Setting clear goals ensures that the consultation remains focused, relevant, and effective.

1. **Identifying Ethical Issues**: The consultation should begin by clearly identifying the ethical issues involved. These may include conflicts between patient autonomy and practitioner beneficence, challenges in adhering to the principles of nonmaleficence, or considerations of fairness and justice in resource allocation.
2. **Defining Desired Outcomes**: Desired outcomes should be articulated to ensure that the consultation addresses the ethical

dilemmas effectively. This may involve ensuring that the patient's autonomy is respected, that the benefits of treatment are maximized while harms are minimized, or that justice is upheld in decision-making processes.

3. **Outlining Steps to Achieve Outcomes**: A structured approach should be developed to achieve the desired outcomes. This involves specifying actions, assigning responsibilities, and setting timelines to ensure that ethical issues are resolved in a timely and efficient manner.

Patient Autonomy and the Role of Informed Consent

Central to the ethics consultation process is the respect for patient autonomy. Informed consent is a fundamental expression of this autonomy, ensuring that patients or their legally established surrogates make healthcare decisions based on a full understanding of their diagnosis, prognosis, treatment options, and the associated benefits and risks. Informed consent must align with the patient's reasonable goals, values, and priorities, and it must be voluntary, free from coercion or undue influence.

- **Role of Surrogates in Decision-Making**: When a patient lacks decisional capacity, surrogate decision-makers are called upon to make decisions on behalf of the patient. Surrogates are expected to use substituted judgment to reflect the patient's known reasonable goals, values, and priorities. In cases where these cannot be determined, surrogates should prioritize beneficence (promoting the patient's well-being) and nonmaleficence (minimize burdens), ensuring compliance with medical standards of care, institutional policies, and legal mandates.

Practitioner Beneficence and Nonmaleficence

Healthcare practitioners are guided by the principles of beneficence and nonmaleficence. These principles require that the care provided promotes the patient's best interests and well-being, while simultaneously minimize burdens. Practitioners must present treatment options that are scientifically validated, aligned with the patient's reasonable goals, values, and priorities, and compliant with medical standards of care.

- **Maximizing Benefits and Minimizing Harm**: In every ethics consultation, practitioners must consider the balance of benefits and risks associated with treatment options. The goal is to maximize patient benefits while minimizing potential harm. Ethics consultations provide a platform for carefully weighing these considerations, ensuring that patient care is not only effective but also ethical.

Public Justice: Ensure Fairness and Equity

The principle of public justice underscores the importance of fairness and equity in healthcare. Ethics consultations play a crucial role in ensuring that all patients are treated fairly and that healthcare decisions do not disproportionately favor or disadvantage any group. This is particularly important in contexts where resources are limited or where systemic disparities may affect the quality of care received.

- **Addressing Broader Social Implications**: Ethics consultations must consider the broader social implications of healthcare decisions. This includes ensuring that policies and practices are in place to address health disparities, promote equitable access to care, and allocate resources fairly. By advocating for public justice, ethics consultations contribute to a more equitable and just healthcare system.

Compliance with Ethical Standards and Legal Mandates

Ensuring compliance with ethical standards and legal mandates is a foundational aspect of the ethics consultation process. Consultations must align with established medical standards of care, institutional policies, and applicable federal and state laws. This alignment ensures that ethical decisions are not only morally sound but also legally defensible.

- **Continuous Education and Ethical Awareness**: The Bioethics Program is committed to fostering continuous education and ethical awareness among healthcare practitioners and ethics consultants. Ongoing education ensures that practitioners are equipped with the knowledge and skills needed to navigate complex ethical dilemmas, uphold ethical standards, and provide care that respects patient autonomy, promotes beneficence, avoids harm, and ensures justice.

Conclusion

The ethics consultation process is a vital tool in addressing ethical dilemmas in healthcare. By adhering to the principles of patient autonomy, practitioner beneficence, nonmaleficence, and public justice, and ensuring compliance with ethical standards and legal mandates, ethics consultations help create a healthcare environment where ethical considerations are integral to every aspect of patient care and decision-making. This approach not only enhances the quality and compassion of patient care but also supports a healthcare system grounded in the highest standards of ethical integrity and justice.

***

Conducting the Ethics Consultation

Gathering Relevant Information

The first step in conducting an ethics consultation is to gather comprehensive and relevant information. This process must ensure that all aspects of the patient's condition, preferences, and the perspectives of involved stakeholders are understood. Ethics consultants must diligently obtain accurate and complete information to form the foundation of a thorough ethical analysis.

Patient's Perspective:

- Ensure that the patient, or their surrogate when the patient lacks decisional capacity, understands their diagnosis and prognosis, the available treatment options (including the option of no treatment), the purpose of each option, and the potential benefits and risks. This comprehensive understanding supports the principle of patient autonomy (informed consent) and aligns with medical standards of care, institutional policies, and legal mandates.

Family's Perspective:

- Engage the patient's family to understand their views and concerns, particularly when acting as surrogates. The family's understanding of the patient's reasonable goals, values, and priorities should guide decision-making in alignment with patient autonomy, nonmaleficence (minimize burdens), and beneficence (maximize benefits).

Healthcare Providers' Perspective:

- Include input from the interprofessional healthcare team to understand the clinical aspects and ethical implications of treatment options. Providers should ensure their recommendations promote the patient's well-being (beneficence) while avoiding unnecessary harm (nonmaleficence), adhering to medical standards of care, institutional policies, and legal mandates.

Engaging with Stakeholders

Ethics consultants must engage all relevant stakeholders, including patients, families, and healthcare providers, through open and respectful dialogue. This engagement should be inclusive and transparent, ensuring that all perspectives are considered and fostering a collaborative approach to ethical decision-making.

1. **Patient and Family Engagement**:
   - Encourage patients and their surrogates to express their understanding, values, and preferences. This aligns with patient autonomy, allowing decisions to reflect the patient's reasonable goals, values, and priorities.
2. **Healthcare Providers Engagement**:
   - Facilitate discussions with healthcare providers to ensure that their clinical insights and ethical considerations align with the principles of beneficence, nonmaleficence, and public justice. This collaboration ensures that all recommendations and actions comply with institutional policies and legal standards.

Analyzing Ethical Dilemmas

The core of the ethics consultation process is to analyze the ethical dilemmas at hand systematically. Ethics consultants should utilize ethical theories and frameworks to balance competing ethical principles and consider the potential consequences of different courses of action.

1. **Patient Autonomy** (Informed Consent):
   - Evaluate the patient's or surrogate's ability to make informed decisions based on a comprehensive understanding of their condition, treatment options, and associated risks and benefits. Decisions should reflect the patient's reasonable goals, values, and priorities.
2. **Practitioner Beneficence** (Maximize Benefits):

- Assess how the proposed treatments can enhance the patient's well-being. Recommendations should aim to maximize benefits in alignment with the patient's reasonable goals, values, and priorities, ensuring compliance with medical standards, institutional policies, and legal requirements.

3. **Practitioner Nonmaleficence** (Minimize Burdens):

   - Identify potential risks and work to minimize harm. Ethical recommendations should prioritize the patient's safety and health, avoiding unnecessary interventions that may cause harm.

4. **Public Justice** (Ensure Fairness):

   - Consider the broader implications of healthcare decisions on society, ensuring that the recommendations uphold fairness and equitable treatment. Align these considerations with institutional policies, medical standards, and legal mandates.

Conclusion

Conducting an effective ethics consultation requires a meticulous and comprehensive approach, beginning with gathering relevant information and engaging with all stakeholders. By prioritizing a thorough understanding of the patient's condition, preferences, and the perspectives of their family and healthcare providers, ethics consultants can ensure that ethical analyses are well-informed and considerate of all involved. This structured process, grounded in the core bioethical principles of patient autonomy, practitioner beneficence, practitioner nonmaleficence, and public justice, facilitates ethical decision-making that respects the patient's reasonable goals, values, and priorities. Through systematic analysis, balanced ethical judgment, and consistent compliance with medical standards, institutional policies, and legal mandates, ethics consultations play a crucial role in enhancing the quality of patient care and fostering an environment of ethical awareness and continuous learning within healthcare institutions.

***

Documentation and Communication

Using SOAP Notes for Ethics Consultations

SOAP (Subjective, Objective, Assessment, Plan) Notes are a critical tool for documenting ethics consultations. They provide a structured format that ensures all relevant information is captured and clearly communicated. The use of SOAP Notes aligns with the Bioethics Program's mission to integrate ethical considerations into patient care by grounding the documentation in the core bioethical principles.

(S) Subjective:

- Document the patient's or surrogate's perspective on the medical condition, diagnosis, and prognosis. Ensure that the patient or surrogate understands the available treatment options, including the option of no treatment, and the purpose of each option. This supports patient autonomy by ensuring informed consent.
- Include statements from the patient or surrogate that articulate the patient's reasonable goals, values, and priorities. This aligns with the principles of beneficence (maximize benefits) and nonmaleficence (minimize burdens), ensuring that care decisions reflect the patient's well-being and risk minimization.

(O) Objective:

- Record objective medical facts, such as diagnosis, clinical observations, and test results. Ensure that these facts are presented clearly and support informed decision-making.
- Include evidence-based information about the benefits and risks of each treatment option, reinforcing the principle of nonmaleficence by providing a basis for minimize burdens and beneficence by promoting the patient's well-being.

(A) Assessment:

- Evaluate the ethical issues identified, ensuring a thorough analysis that balances the bioethical principles of patient autonomy, practitioner beneficence, practitioner nonmaleficence, and public justice. Assess the patient's capacity to make informed decisions or the surrogate's ability to provide substituted judgment when necessary.
- Clearly articulate the ethical dilemmas and provide a reasoned assessment that considers the patient's reasonable goals, values, and priorities, while ensuring adherence to medical standards of care, institutional policies, and legal mandates.

(P) Plan:

- Develop a plan that outlines the recommended course of action, specifying how the bioethical principles have been weighed and balanced. Ensure that the plan includes steps for communicating findings and recommendations to all stakeholders.
- Address the need for ongoing education and dialogue with healthcare practitioners to foster ethical awareness and understanding, as mandated by the Bioethics Program's mission.

Writing Clear and Comprehensive Reports

Ethics consultants must prepare reports that summarize their findings and recommendations concisely and comprehensively. These reports should be organized in a way that is accessible to all stakeholders, ensuring that the recommendations are understood and can be implemented effectively.

Clarity and Structure:

- Use clear language that avoids jargon and is understandable to non-medical stakeholders, ensuring that the report is accessible to all involved parties.

- Organize the report logically, starting with a summary of the ethical issues, followed by a detailed analysis, and concluding with specific recommendations. This structure should reflect the SOAP framework to ensure consistency and clarity.

Inclusivity and Transparency:

- Include input from all relevant stakeholders, such as patients, surrogates, family members, and healthcare providers, ensuring that their perspectives are considered and documented.
- Highlight the ethical reasoning behind each recommendation, ensuring transparency and building trust in the consultation process. This approach aligns with the Bioethics Program's vision of fostering an ethical culture and ensuring that all decisions are guided by the principles of fairness and public justice.

Communicating Findings and Recommendations

Effective communication is essential for the successful implementation of ethics consultation findings and recommendations. Ethics consultants must present their conclusions clearly and persuasively, addressing any concerns or questions from stakeholders to ensure the ethical issues are resolved satisfactorily.

Effective Communication:

- Communicate findings and recommendations verbally and in writing, ensuring that all stakeholders, including patients, surrogates, and healthcare providers, understand the ethical analysis and proposed actions.
- Use language that respects the patient's and surrogate's perspectives, values, and cultural backgrounds, promoting an inclusive approach to ethical decision-making.

Addressing Concerns:

- Be prepared to address concerns or objections from stakeholders, providing clear explanations of how the recommendations align with the patient's reasonable goals, values, and priorities and the core bioethical principles.
- Encourage dialogue and feedback from stakeholders to refine recommendations and ensure that they are practical, ethically sound, and in the patient's best interests.

Conclusion

Incorporating a structured approach like SOAP Notes into ethics consultations is fundamental to ensuring that ethical considerations are effectively integrated into patient care. This structured documentation and communication framework not only provides clarity and consistency but also ensures that the core bioethical principles of patient autonomy, beneficence, nonmaleficence, and public justice are systematically addressed. By using SOAP Notes, ethics consultants can clearly document the ethical dilemmas, articulate the reasoning behind their recommendations, and foster a transparent dialogue among all stakeholders. This approach supports the Bioethics Program's mission of promoting ethical awareness and sound decision-making, ultimately enhancing the quality, compassion, and fairness of patient care.

***

Follow-Up and Evaluation

Ensuring Implementation of Recommendations

After an ethics consultation, it is crucial to ensure that the recommendations are implemented effectively to maximize the patient's best interests. This involves close collaboration with healthcare teams to integrate ethical recommendations into patient care plans, ensuring alignment with the bioethical principles of patient autonomy (informed consent), practitioner beneficence (maximize benefits), practitioner nonmaleficence (minimize burdens), and public justice (ensure fairness).

Implementation Strategies:

- **Patient Autonomy** (Informed Consent): Ensure that patients or their surrogates have a clear understanding of the recommendations and how they align with the patient's reasonable goals, values, and priorities. Confirm that patients or surrogates understand the diagnosis, prognosis, available options (including the option of no treatment), the purpose of each option, and the potential benefits and risks, thereby supporting informed consent.
- **Practitioner Beneficence** (Maximize Benefits): Advocate for care plans that enhance the patient's well-being. Engage with healthcare providers to prioritize treatment options that promote good outcomes, considering the patient's reasonable goals, values, and priorities. Recommendations should be in accordance with established medical standards of care, institutional policies, and legal mandates.
- **Practitioner Nonmaleficence** (Minimize Burdens): Work to minimize any potential harm to the patient by avoiding unnecessary or overly aggressive treatments. Ensure that the implementation of recommendations adheres to safety

protocols and ethical guidelines, protecting the patient from harm.

- **Public Justice** (Ensure Fairness): Address any barriers to implementing recommendations that may arise from resource limitations or institutional constraints. Advocate for fair and equitable treatment, ensuring that the patient's access to care is not compromised and that decisions are made transparently and ethically.

Monitoring Outcomes and Impact

Monitoring the outcomes of ethics consultation recommendations is essential to assess their effectiveness and impact on patient care and ethical decision-making. This process ensures that ethical considerations continue to guide healthcare practices and supports continuous improvement.

Outcome Assessment:

- **Patient Autonomy** (Informed Consent): Evaluate whether patients or surrogates felt adequately informed and supported in their decision-making process. Gather feedback on their understanding of the recommendations and their perceived alignment with their reasonable goals, values, and priorities.
- **Practitioner Beneficence** (Maximize Benefits): Assess the health outcomes resulting from the implemented recommendations. Measure improvements in patient well-being and satisfaction, ensuring that the care provided is consistent with the principles of beneficence.
- **Practitioner Nonmaleficence** (Minimize Burdens): Monitor for any adverse events or harm that may have occurred as a result of the implemented recommendations. Use this data to refine future recommendations, ensuring that ethical guidelines are effectively preventing harm.
- **Public Justice** (Ensure Fairness): Review the fairness of the recommendations' implementation. Consider whether all

patients had equal access to ethics consultations and whether the recommendations were applied consistently across similar cases. This helps ensure that public justice is upheld.

Continuous Quality Improvement in Ethics Consultation

Continuous quality improvement (CQI) is integral to the effectiveness of ethics consultation services. By regularly reviewing and refining consultation processes, ethics consultants can remain responsive to the evolving needs of patients, families, and healthcare providers.

CQI Strategies:

- **Feedback and Review:** Establish mechanisms for gathering feedback from patients, surrogates, healthcare providers, and other stakeholders involved in the ethics consultation. Use this feedback to identify areas for improvement and to ensure that the consultation process aligns with the Bioethics Program's mission and vision.
- **Training and Education:** Provide ongoing training and education for ethics consultants and healthcare providers to keep them informed about developments in bioethics, legal mandates, and institutional policies. This helps maintain high standards of ethical awareness and decision-making.
- **Ethical Reflection and Dialogue:** Promote a culture of ethical reflection and open dialogue within the healthcare institution. Encourage practitioners to regularly discuss ethical challenges and share insights, fostering a collaborative approach to ethical decision-making.
- **Policy Review and Development:** Regularly review and update institutional policies related to ethics consultation. Ensure that these policies reflect current ethical standards, legal requirements, and best practices, supporting the principles of patient autonomy, practitioner beneficence, practitioner nonmaleficence, and public justice.

Conclusion

Effective follow-up and evaluation are vital components of the ethics consultation process, ensuring that recommendations are not only implemented but also achieve their intended outcomes. By focusing on patient autonomy (informed consent), practitioner beneficence (maximize benefits), practitioner nonmaleficence (minimize burdens), and public justice (ensure fairness), ethics consultants can guide the integration of ethical considerations into patient care, improving both the quality of care and the decision-making process. Monitoring outcomes and engaging in continuous quality improvement help maintain high standards of ethical practice, supporting a healthcare environment that is responsive to the needs of patients, families, and providers. Through these efforts, the Bioethics Program upholds its commitment to ethical reflection, education, and the consistent application of ethical principles, fostering a culture of integrity and compassion in healthcare.

***

The following forms, templates, and checklists provide the structured tools necessary to effectively conduct, document, and follow up on ethics consultations. They will help ensure that the ethics consultation process is thorough, consistent, and aligned with the highest standards of ethical practice.

***

2.1 Ethics Consultation Request Form

Purpose: To formally request an ethics consultation, capturing essential information to facilitate a prompt and effective response.

Date of Request: ______________________________

Time of Request: ______________________________

Patient Information

- **Patient Name**: ______________________________
- **Date of Birth**: ______________________________
- **Medical Record Number**: ______________________

Requestor Information

- **Name**: ______________________________
- **Role/Title**: ______________________________
- **Department**: ______________________________
- **Contact Information**: ______________________

Reason for Consultation

- **Primary Ethical Issue(s)**: [Brief description of the ethical issue(s) prompting the consultation]
- **Specific Questions or Concerns**: [List any specific questions or concerns that need to be addressed]

Involved Parties

- ☐ **Patient**:
- ☐ **Family Members**: [List names if applicable]
- ☐ **Healthcare Team Members**: [List names and roles]
- ☐ **Others** (e.g., legal, social work, clergy): [List names and roles]

Urgency of Consultation

- ☐ **Immediate** (within hours)
- ☐ **Soon** (within 24-48 hours)
- ☐ **Routine** (within a few days)

Initial Actions Taken

- [Summary of any actions taken by the requestor prior to submitting the request]

Consultant Assigned: ___________________________________

Date/Time of Assignment: _______________________________

***

2.2 Ethics Consultation Preparation Checklist

Purpose: To guide ethics consultants in preparing for a consultation by ensuring all relevant information is gathered and considered.

Pre-Consultation Information Gathering

- ☐ Review Patient's Medical Records
- ☐ Identify Advance Directives (if any)
- ☐ Gather Input from Healthcare Team
- ☐ Contact Family Members (if applicable)
- ☐ Review Relevant Legal/Institutional Policies
- ☐ Assess Cultural/Religious Considerations

Stakeholder Engagement

- ☐ Schedule Initial Meeting with Stakeholders
- ☐ Ensure All Relevant Parties are Informed and Prepared
- ☐ Plan for Confidentiality and Sensitive Information Handling

Setting Goals and Objectives

- ☐ Define Key Ethical Issues
- ☐ Outline Desired Outcomes of the Consultation
- ☐ Determine the Steps to Achieve These Outcomes

Consultation Logistics

- ☐ Confirm Time and Location of Consultation
- ☐ Prepare Necessary Documentation Tools (e.g., SOAP Notes)
- ☐ Arrange for Follow-Up Sessions if Required

***

2.3 SOAP Notes

Purpose: To provide a comprehensive and structured format for documenting ethics consultations using the SOAP (Subjective, Objective, Assessment, Plan) method.

Consultation Date: [Date]
Consultant: [Name/Title]
Patient/Case ID: [ID]
Department: [Department Name]

---

1. (S) Subjective

Patient's Perspective

- **Narrative**: Document the patient's understanding of their medical condition, goals, values, and concerns.

  Open-ended Questions:

  - "Can you tell me about your understanding of your current medical condition?"
  - "What are your goals and priorities regarding your treatment?"
  - "How do you feel about the proposed medical interventions?"
  - "Are there any specific concerns or values that are particularly important to you in making healthcare decisions?"

Family's Perspective

- **Narrative**: Document the family's understanding, goals, and concerns regarding the patient's condition and treatment.

  Open-ended Questions:

  - "Can you share your thoughts and concerns about your loved one's medical condition and treatment?"
  - "What are your goals and priorities for your loved one's care?"
  - "How do you think your loved one feels about their current situation and the proposed treatments?"

- "How do you think your loved one's values and priorities should guide the decisions being made?"

PRACTITIONERS' PERSPECTIVE

- **Narrative**: Document the practitioners' views on the medical condition, treatment plan, and ethical considerations.

  Open-ended Questions:

  - "Can you explain the medical condition and proposed treatment plan?"
  - "What do you see as the primary benefits and risks of the proposed interventions?"
  - "How do you incorporate the patient's values and preferences into the treatment plan?"
  - "Is the proposed treatment plan in alignment with current healthcare standards of care, institutional policies, and professional guidelines?"
  - "How do you ensure that the treatment plan reflects the patient's reasonable goals, values, and priorities?"

---

2. (O) Objective

Medical Facts:

- **Summary**: Provide an overview of the patient's medical condition, diagnosis, and prognosis.
- **Clinical Data**: Include relevant medical history, current treatments, and proposed interventions.
- **Observations**: Note any observations related to the patient's condition and interactions with staff.
- **Alignment**: Ensure that all medical facts align with current medical standards of care.

---

3. (A) Assessment

Ethical Issues Identified:

- **Patient Autonomy** (informed consent):
  - Assess the patient's capacity to make informed decisions.

  - Document the information provided to the patient about treatment options.
- **Practitioner Beneficence** (maximize benefits)**:**
  - Evaluate the potential benefits of the proposed interventions.
- **Practitioner Nonmaleficence** (minimize burdens)**:**
  - Identify potential risks and harms associated with the treatments.
- **Public Justice** (ensure fairness)**:**
  - Consider fairness in the allocation of resources and treatment options.
- **Alignment with Medical Standards of Care:**
  - Ensure proposed treatment plans adhere to current medical healthcare standards.
- **Patient's Reasonable Goals, Values, and Priorities:**
  - Ensure these are central to the ethical analysis and treatment plan.
- **Compliance with Professional, Institutional, State, and Federal Standards:**
  - Verify that the treatment plan complies with relevant laws, policies, and social expectations.

---

4. (P) Plan

Ethical Recommendations:

- **Steps**: Outline specific steps to address the identified ethical issues.
- **Communication**: Include a plan for further communication with the patient, family, and practitioners.
- **Decisions**: Document any decisions made during the consultation.

Follow-up:

- **Meetings**: Schedule follow-up meetings to reassess the situation and ensure implementation of ethical recommendations.

- **Responsibilities**: Assign responsibilities to team members for monitoring the patient's condition and ethical aspects of care.

Documentation:

- **EHR**: Ensure all discussions, decisions, and plans are thoroughly documented in the patient's Electronic Health Record (EHR).
- **Alignment**: Confirm that documentation reflects alignment with current healthcare standards, the patient's reasonable goals, values, and priorities, and compliance with professional, institutional, state, and federal standards.

Signature: [Consultant's Signature]
Date: [Date]

***

2.4 SOAP Notes—Cue Card

(S) Subjective

Patient:
- Understand condition?
- Goals and priorities?
- Feelings about treatment?
- Important values/concerns?

Family:
- Thoughts/concerns?
- Goals for loved one?
- Loved one's values/priorities?

Practitioners:
- Condition/treatment explanation?
- Benefits/risks?
- Alignment with standards of care?
- Patient's values/preferences?

(O) Objective

- Medical condition/prognosis
- Treatments/interventions
- Standards of care/compliance

(A) Assessment

Ethical analysis:
- Ethical issues (Autonomy, Beneficence, Nonmaleficence, Justice)
- Alignment with medical standards of care
- Patient's Reasonable Goals, Values, and Priorities
- Compliance with Professional, Institutional, State, and Federal mandates

---

(P) Plan

Action steps:
- Address issues
- Communicate plan
- Document decisions
- Follow-up schedule
- Compliance with medical standards of care

***

2.5 Ethics Consultation Follow-Up Checklist

Purpose: To ensure that the recommendations from an ethics consultation are implemented and to monitor their outcomes.

Implementation of Recommendations

- ☐ Confirm Recommendations are Integrated into Care Plan
- ☐ Address Any Barriers to Implementation
- ☐ Ensure Stakeholders are Informed and Aligned

Monitoring and Evaluation

- ☐ Monitor Patient Outcomes Related to the Consultation
- ☐ Evaluate the Impact on Ethical Decision-Making
- ☐ Gather Feedback from Stakeholders on the Consultation Process

Continuous Quality Improvement

- ☐ Review and Analyze Consultation Outcomes
- ☐ Identify Areas for Process Improvement
- ☐ Document Lessons Learned for Future Consultations

Final Documentation

- ☐ Update SOAP Notes with Follow-Up Information
- ☐ Ensure All Documentation is Complete and Accessible
- ☐ Schedule Additional Follow-Up if Needed

Consultant Name: ____
Date/Time Completed: ____________________________________

***

2.6 Ethics Consultation Report Template

Purpose: To create a clear, comprehensive, and concise report summarizing the ethics consultation and its outcomes.

Patient Name: ______________________________
Date of Birth: ______________________________
Medical Record Number: ______________________
Consultation Date: __________________________

Consultation Summary

- **Reason for Consultation**: [Summary of the ethical issue(s) and reason for the consultation]
- **Stakeholders Involved**: [List of individuals and their roles in the consultation]

Ethical Analysis

- **Key Ethical Issues**: [Detailed analysis of the ethical dilemmas involved]
- **Application of Ethical Principles**: [How core ethical principles were applied in the analysis]
- **Consultant's Assessment**: [Summary of the consultant's ethical assessment and rationale]

Recommendations

- **Specific Recommendations**: [List the recommendations provided to the healthcare team and/or family]
- **Rationale for Recommendations**: [Explanation of the reasoning behind the recommendations]

Follow-Up Plan

- **Next Steps**: [Any additional actions required, including follow-up consultations]
- **Monitoring and Evaluation**: [Plans for monitoring the outcomes and impact of the recommendations]

Consultant Name: ______________________________________

Date/Time Completed: __________________________________

***

Review Questions

True/False Questions:

1. Ethics consultations are initiated only when there are legal disputes between patients and healthcare providers.
True or False?

2. Gathering relevant information is an essential step in conducting an ethics consultation.
True or False?

3. SOAP Notes are used to document ethics consultations because they provide a structured format for recording the process.
True or False?

4. Ethics consultants do not need to engage with patients' families during the consultation process.
True or False?

5. Continuous quality improvement is not necessary for maintaining the effectiveness of ethics consultation services.
True or False?

Multiple-Choice Questions:

6. Which of the following is a primary goal of an ethics consultation?
a) To reduce healthcare costs
b) To enhance the quality of patient care by integrating ethical considerations
c) To enforce legal standards in healthcare
d) To provide medical treatment options

7. What does the 'A' in SOAP Notes stand for?
a) Analysis
b) Assessment
c) Application
d) Action

Clinical Vignettes:

8. **Scenario:** Mrs. Lee, an elderly patient, has advanced dementia and no advance directives. Her children disagree on whether to continue aggressive treatment or transition to palliative care. The healthcare team is also unsure how to proceed. What is the best course of action?
a) Continue aggressive treatment indefinitely
b) Withdraw aggressive treatment immediately
c) Involve an ethics consultant to facilitate discussions and reach a consensus
d) Make a decision based on the healthcare team's majority opinion

9. **Scenario:** John, a young adult, refuses a recommended surgery due to his fear of anesthesia. The interprofessional healthcare team believes the surgery is necessary for his health. What is the best course of action?
a) Proceed with the surgery against his wishes
b) Respect his decision without further discussion
c) Call an ethics consultant to mediate and explore a respectful solution
d) Transfer him to another hospital

10. **Scenario:** Dr. Smith, a physician, is faced with a dilemma where a patient requests an experimental treatment that is not yet approved. The patient is fully informed of the risks but is desperate for any possible benefit. What is the best course of action?
a) Provide the experimental treatment without further consideration
b) Deny the request outright
c) Seek an ethics consultation to analyze the ethical implications and provide recommendations
d) Ask the patient to find another doctor willing to take the risk

Correct Answers:

1. False (Ethics consultations are initiated to address complex ethical issues in patient care, not just legal disputes. They can involve a wide range of ethical dilemmas, including conflicts between patient wishes and medical recommendations, uncertainties about appropriate courses of action, and disputes among patients, families, and healthcare providers.)
2. True
3. True
4. False (Ethics consultants often engage with patients' families during the consultation process to ensure that all perspectives are considered and to facilitate discussions that respect the values and wishes of the patient and their family.)
5. False (Continuous quality improvement is essential for maintaining the effectiveness of ethics consultation services, ensuring that the process remains responsive to the needs of patients, families, and healthcare providers, and that it keeps pace with developments in the field of bioethics.)
6. b) To enhance the quality of patient care by integrating ethical considerations
7. b) Assessment
8. c) Involve an ethics consultant to facilitate discussions and reach a consensus
9. c) Call an ethics consultant to mediate and explore a respectful

solution
10. c) Seek an ethics consultation to analyze the ethical implications and provide recommendations

***

Further Readings and References

- Aulisio, M. P., Arnold, R. M., & Youngner, S. J. (2000). "*Health Care Ethics Consultation: Nature, Goals, and Competencies.*" In J. Sugarman & D. P. Sulmasy (Eds.), Methods in Medical Ethics (pp. 180-196). Georgetown University Press.
  - *This comprehensive overview discusses the nature and goals of healthcare ethics consultation, providing essential information on the competencies required for effective practice.*
- Jonsen, A. R., Siegler, M., & Winslade, W. J. (2015). Clinical Ethics: A Practical Approach to Ethical Decisions in Clinical Medicine (8th ed.). McGraw-Hill Education.
  - *A practical guide addressing ethical dilemmas in clinical practice, with case studies and frameworks for decision-making.*
- American Society for Bioethics and Humanities (ASBH). (2011). Core Competencies for Healthcare Ethics Consultation. ASBH.
  - *This document outlines the essential skills and knowledge required for healthcare ethics consultants, emphasizing the role of ethics consultation in clinical practice.*
- Beauchamp, T. L., & Childress, J. F. (2019). Principles of Biomedical Ethics (8th ed.). Oxford University Press.
  - *This foundational text provides an in-depth discussion of the four principles of biomedical ethics: autonomy, beneficence, nonmaleficence, and justice.*
- Fins, J. J., & Bacchetta, M. D. (1995). "*Framing the Clinical Ethics Case Consultation: A Pedagogical and Problem-Oriented Approach.*" *Journal of Clinical Ethics*, 6(3), 239-251.
  - *This article offers a pedagogical approach to conducting ethics consultations, focusing on case framing and problem-solving strategies.*

- Quill, T. E., & Cassel, C. K. (1995). "*Nonabandonment: A Central Obligation for Physicians." Annals of Internal Medicine*, 122(5), 368-374.
  - *An article discussing the ethical obligation of nonabandonment in the physician-patient relationship, relevant to the role of ethics consultants in ensuring continuous care.*
- Grady, C. (2010). "*Do IRBs Protect Human Research Participants?*" *JAMA*, 304(10), 1122-1123.
  - *This article discusses the role of Institutional Review Boards (IRBs) in protecting human research participants, relevant to the ethics consultation process in research settings.*
- Dubler, N. N., & Liebman, C. B. (2011). Bioethics Mediation: A Guide to Shaping Shared Solutions. Vanderbilt University Press.
  - *A guide on using mediation techniques in bioethics consultations to shape shared solutions and resolve conflicts.*
- Pellegrino, E. D., & Thomasma, D. C. (1993). The Virtues in Medical Practice. Oxford University Press.
  - *A philosophical exploration of the virtues essential to medical practice, including the role of ethics consultation in promoting virtuous behavior in healthcare.*
- Truog, R. D., et al. (2008). "*Recommendations for End-of-Life Care in the Intensive Care Unit: A Consensus Statement by the American College of Critical Care Medicine." Critical Care Medicine*, 36(3), 953-963.
  - *Consensus recommendations on end-of-life care in the ICU, highlighting the ethical considerations and the role of ethics consultation in decision-making.*

***

Part III: Practical Skills for Ethics Consultants

Communication and Mediation Skills

Active Listening and Empathy

Active listening and empathy are fundamental skills for ethics consultants, essential for ensuring that all stakeholders' concerns and perspectives are understood and respected. These skills support patient autonomy by creating an environment where patients and their surrogates feel heard and valued, facilitating informed consent and decision-making based on their reasonable goals, values, and priorities.

- **Patient Autonomy** (informed consent): Ethics consultants must use active listening to ensure that patients or their surrogates fully understand their diagnosis, prognosis, available treatment options, the purpose of each option, and the associated benefits and risks. This understanding is crucial for informed consent, allowing patients to make decisions that reflect their reasonable goals, values, and priorities.
- **Empathy:** Demonstrating empathy helps ethics consultants build trust and rapport with stakeholders. By understanding and sharing the feelings of others, consultants can more effectively address emotional concerns, ensuring that ethical discussions remain supportive and respectful. This approach promotes the principles of beneficence (maximize benefits) and nonmaleficence (minimize burdens) by fostering a compassionate care environment.

Facilitating Difficult Conversations

Ethics consultants often facilitate conversations about sensitive and emotionally charged issues, such as end-of-life care, refusal of treatment, or conflicts between patient and family wishes. Effective facilitation involves creating a safe space for open dialogue, guiding discussions to ensure that all voices are heard, and helping participants find common ground.

- **Creating a Safe Environment:** Establish a respectful and supportive atmosphere where participants feel comfortable expressing their views and concerns. This environment supports patient autonomy by allowing patients and surrogates to voice their preferences and values freely.
- **Guiding the Discussion:** Use ethical principles as a framework to guide conversations. Highlight how different perspectives align with or challenge the principles of patient autonomy (informed consent), practitioner beneficence (maximize benefits), practitioner nonmaleficence (minimize burdens), and public justice (ensure fairness). Help participants understand the implications of their choices, ensuring that the discussions lead to well-informed decisions.
- **Managing Emotions:** Be prepared to address strong emotions that may arise. Use empathy and active listening to acknowledge feelings and validate concerns, fostering a constructive dialogue that focuses on finding ethically sound solutions.

Conflict Resolution and Mediation

Conflict resolution and mediation skills are essential for ethics consultants when disputes arise among patients, families, and healthcare providers. These skills help identify the underlying causes of conflict, develop strategies for resolution, and promote collaborative decision-making.

- **Identifying Underlying Issues:** Use active listening and empathetic engagement to uncover the root causes of conflict. Understanding these issues is crucial for addressing them effectively and aligning solutions with the bioethical principles.

- **Developing Resolution Strategies:** Create strategies that consider the reasonable goals, values, and priorities of all parties involved. Ensure that proposed solutions adhere to the principles of patient autonomy (informed consent), practitioner beneficence (maximize benefits), practitioner nonmaleficence (minimize burdens), and public justice (ensure fairness). Aim for resolutions that maximize patient well-being and minimize harm while ensure fairness and equity.
- **Fostering Collaboration:** Encourage cooperation among patients, surrogates, families, and healthcare providers. Emphasize the importance of working together to achieve the patient's best interests, guided by ethical principles and in compliance with medical standards of care, institutional policies, and legal mandates.

Mastering communication and mediation skills is crucial for ethics consultants, enabling them to navigate the complex ethical dilemmas that arise in healthcare settings. By focusing on active listening, empathy, effective facilitation, and conflict resolution, consultants can ensure that ethical considerations are thoughtfully integrated into patient care. This approach not only upholds the core bioethical principles of patient autonomy, practitioner beneficence, practitioner nonmaleficence, and public justice but also fosters an environment of trust, respect, and collaboration. Through these efforts, the Bioethics Program continues to support ethically sound decision-making, enhancing the quality and compassion of patient care.

***

Analytical and Critical Thinking Skills

Applying Ethical Theories and Principles

Ethics consultants must be proficient in applying ethical theories and principles to real-world situations, ensuring that their analyses align with the core bioethical principles of patient autonomy (informed consent), practitioner beneficence (maximize benefits), practitioner nonmaleficence (minimize burdens), and public justice (ensure fairness). This skill involves understanding the nuances of different ethical frameworks, such as virtue ethics, deontology, and consequentialism, and using these frameworks to analyze and resolve ethical dilemmas. Consultants must critically evaluate the strengths and limitations of each approach and apply them appropriately within specific contexts.

- **Patient Autonomy** (Informed Consent): In every ethical analysis, emphasize the patient's right to informed consent. Ensure that patients or their surrogates are fully informed about their medical condition, available treatment options, and the risks and benefits associated with each option. Ethical theories should support decision-making that reflects the patient's reasonable goals, values, and priorities.
- **Practitioner Beneficence** (Maximize Benefits): Use ethical theories to advocate for actions that enhance the patient's well-being. The application of these theories should promote the maximization of benefits to the patient, ensuring that the care provided aligns with the patient's reasonable goals, values, and priorities.
- **Practitioner Nonmaleficence** (Minimize Burdens): Evaluate ethical dilemmas to minimize harm. Ethical theories should help identify potential risks and guide the development of

recommendations that protect the patient's safety and health, avoiding unnecessary or harmful interventions.

- **Public Justice** (Ensure Fairness): Apply ethical principles to ensure fairness and equity in decision-making. Ethical theories should help balance individual patient needs with broader societal considerations, promoting fair treatment and adherence to institutional policies and legal mandates.

Systematic Approaches to Ethical Analysis

A systematic approach to ethical analysis ensures that all relevant factors are considered in the decision-making process. Ethics consultants should utilize structured tools and methodologies such as the Think, Assess, and Conclude (TAC) method, to guide their analysis and develop well-founded recommendations that can then me entered in the Electronic Health Records (EHR) using, for example, the SOAP Notes structure that most healthcare professionals are used to.

- **Structured Analysis:** Utilize tools that allow for a comprehensive review of the patient's medical facts, patient preferences, quality of life considerations, and contextual features. This approach ensures that ethical analysis is thorough, consistent, and transparent, supporting patient autonomy by thoroughly exploring the patient's reasonable goals, values, and priorities.
- **Consistency and Transparency:** Apply consistent ethical methodologies across cases to ensure fairness and equity. By maintaining transparency in the decision-making process, ethics consultants uphold public justice and build trust among patients, families, and healthcare providers.

Decision-Making Models and Tools

Ethics consultants should be familiar with various decision-making models and tools that aid in ethical analysis. These models provide structured frameworks for evaluating options, balancing competing principles, and making informed decisions. Decision-making tools help clarify complex issues, facilitate consensus, and support ethical decision-making.

- **Balancing Principles:** Use decision-making models to weigh the principles of autonomy, beneficence, nonmaleficence, and public justice. These models should guide consultants in developing recommendations that align with the Bioethics Program's mission and vision, ensuring compliance with medical standards, institutional policies, and legal mandates.
- **Facilitating Consensus:** Implement decision-making tools that foster collaboration among patients, surrogates, healthcare providers, and other stakeholders. By promoting open dialogue and understanding, these tools support informed consent and help achieve ethically sound and mutually agreeable solutions.

Conclusion

Developing strong analytical and critical thinking skills is essential for ethics consultants, enabling them to navigate the complexities of ethical dilemmas in healthcare. By applying ethical theories and principles systematically and utilizing structured decision-making models, consultants can ensure that their recommendations align with the core bioethical principles and the Bioethics Program's mission and vision. This approach not only promotes ethical decision-making that respects informed consent, enhances well-being, minimizes harm, and ensures fairness but also fosters a culture of ethical awareness and continuous learning within healthcare institutions.

***

Cultural Competence and Sensitivity

Understanding Cultural Differences in Healthcare

Cultural competence is a cornerstone of effective ethics consultation in diverse healthcare settings, aligning closely with the core bioethical principles of patient autonomy (informed consent), practitioner beneficence (maximize benefits), practitioner nonmaleficence (minimize burdens), and public justice (ensure fairness). Ethics consultants must understand and respect cultural differences, recognizing how cultural values and beliefs influence patient care decisions. Developing cultural competence involves being aware of one's own cultural biases, learning about the cultures of others, and adapting communication and consultation approaches accordingly.

- **Patient Autonomy** (Informed Consent): Understanding cultural differences enhances the ability of ethics consultants to ensure informed consent. Consultants must be able to explain diagnoses, treatment options, and their purposes in a way that resonates with the cultural context of the patient or surrogate. This approach ensures that patients or surrogates can make decisions that truly reflect their reasonable goals, values, and priorities.
- **Practitioner Beneficence** (Maximize Benefits): By appreciating cultural differences, ethics consultants can advocate for care plans that enhance patient well-being. Recognizing and respecting cultural values can lead to more culturally appropriate care that aligns with the patient's best interests, thereby promoting good outcomes.
- **Practitioner Nonmaleficence** (Minimize Burdens): Sensitivity to cultural differences is crucial in avoiding potential harm. Misunderstandings or disregard for cultural

beliefs can lead to unnecessary harm or distress. Ethics consultants should strive to ensure that recommendations are culturally appropriate, minimizing any risk of harm.

- **Public Justice** (Ensure Fairness): Cultural competence supports fairness and equitable treatment in healthcare. By respecting diverse cultural values and beliefs, ethics consultants contribute to a healthcare environment where all patients are treated with respect and dignity, supporting the principle of public justice.

Respecting Diverse Values and Beliefs

Ethics consultants must be sensitive to the diverse values and beliefs of patients and their families, finding ways to honor these values in the decision-making process. Respecting diverse perspectives builds trust and ensures that ethical recommendations are culturally appropriate.

- **Building Trust:** Demonstrating respect for diverse values and beliefs helps build trust with patients and their families. Trust is essential for effective communication and ethical decision-making, fostering an environment where patients and surrogates feel comfortable expressing their goals, values, and priorities.
- **Honoring Cultural Perspectives:** Ethics consultants should strive to incorporate patients' cultural beliefs into their recommendations, aligning ethical analyses with the patient's worldview. This approach promotes patient autonomy by ensuring that decisions are informed and reflective of the patient's cultural context.

Strategies for Culturally Sensitive Consultations

Culturally sensitive consultations require tailored approaches that consider the cultural context of ethical issues. Ethics consultants should develop strategies to engage effectively with diverse populations, ensuring that their recommendations are culturally appropriate and respectful.

- **Tailored Communication:** Use culturally appropriate communication styles that resonate with the patient's or surrogate's cultural background. This may involve using culturally specific metaphors, avoiding certain expressions, or adjusting communication based on cultural norms.
- **Involving Cultural Mediators:** When necessary, involve cultural mediators or interpreters who can bridge communication gaps and provide insights into cultural nuances. This ensures that ethics consultations are conducted in a manner that respects the patient's cultural background, supporting informed consent and ethical decision-making.
- **Integrating Cultural Values into Ethical Analysis:** Consider cultural values as part of the ethical analysis. This integration ensures that recommendations are not only ethically sound but also culturally relevant, thereby enhancing patient well-being and minimizing harm.

Conclusion

Cultural competence and sensitivity are essential for ethics consultants, enabling them to provide ethical guidance that respects and honors the diverse cultural values and beliefs of patients. By understanding cultural differences, respecting diverse perspectives, and developing strategies for culturally sensitive consultations, ethics consultants can uphold the bioethical principles of patient autonomy (informed consent), practitioner beneficence (maximize benefits), practitioner nonmaleficence (minimize burdens), and public justice (ensure fairness). This approach ensures that ethical recommendations are not only aligned with the Bioethics Program's mission and vision but also contribute to a healthcare environment that values and respects cultural diversity, promoting equity and fairness in patient care.

***

Interprofessional Collaboration

Working with Healthcare Teams

Effective ethics consultation requires collaboration with interprofessional healthcare teams, ensuring that ethical considerations are thoroughly integrated into patient care. By fostering strong working relationships with team members, ethics consultants can facilitate open communication and shared decision-making, aligning with the bioethical principles of patient autonomy (informed consent), practitioner beneficence (maximize benefits), practitioner nonmaleficence (minimize burdens), and public justice (ensure fairness).

- **Patient Autonomy** (Informed Consent): Collaboration ensures that patients or their surrogates receive consistent and accurate information about their diagnosis, prognosis, and available treatment options. By working closely with healthcare teams, ethics consultants help ensure that the patient's reasonable goals, values, and priorities are understood and respected, facilitating informed consent.
- **Practitioner Beneficence** (Maximize Benefits): Ethics consultants collaborate with healthcare providers to identify and promote treatment options that enhance patient well-being. This joint effort helps ensure that the care plans developed are in the best interest of the patient, reflecting the principles of beneficence and aligning with medical standards, institutional policies, and legal requirements.
- **Practitioner Nonmaleficence** (Minimize Burdens): Collaborative efforts help identify potential risks and avoid unnecessary harm to the patient. By bringing together diverse expertise, healthcare teams can develop care plans that minimize risks and adhere to ethical and safety protocols.

- **Public Justice** (Ensure Fairness): Collaboration among healthcare teams supports fair and equitable treatment of all patients. By integrating diverse perspectives, ethics consultants help ensure that ethical recommendations consider the broader implications of healthcare decisions on society, ensure fairness and justice.

Building Trust and Rapport with Stakeholders

Building trust and rapport with stakeholders is crucial for the success of ethics consultations. Ethics consultants should be transparent, respectful, and responsive to the needs and concerns of all parties involved, demonstrating integrity and maintaining confidentiality.

- **Trust and Transparency:** Establishing trust requires ethics consultants to be consistently reliable and honest in their communications. Transparency in ethical decision-making processes builds confidence among patients, families, and healthcare providers, ensuring that all parties feel respected and understood.
- **Respect and Responsiveness:** Ethics consultants should actively listen to and respect the views of all stakeholders, including patients, surrogates, and healthcare team members. By being responsive to their concerns and needs, consultants can build rapport and facilitate a collaborative approach to ethical decision-making.
- **Confidentiality:** Maintaining confidentiality is essential for building trust. Ethics consultants must ensure that sensitive information is handled appropriately, respecting patient privacy and fostering a secure environment for ethical discussions.

Navigating Interprofessional Dynamics

Navigating the dynamics of interprofessional relationships can be challenging but is essential for effective ethics consultation. Ethics consultants must be skilled in managing power dynamics, addressing conflicts, and fostering a collaborative team environment.

- **Understanding Roles and Perspectives:** Ethics consultants should seek to understand the roles, expertise, and perspectives of different healthcare team members. This understanding promotes mutual respect and helps consultants facilitate interactions that are constructive and respectful of each professional's contribution to patient care.
- **Addressing Conflicts:** When conflicts arise, ethics consultants play a critical role in mediating and resolving disagreements. By using ethical principles to guide discussions, consultants can help align the team's actions with the patient's best interests, promoting beneficence and nonmaleficence.
- **Fostering Collaboration:** Ethics consultants should encourage a team-based approach to ethical decision-making. By promoting open dialogue and mutual respect, consultants help create a collaborative environment where the principles of patient autonomy (informed consent), practitioner beneficence (maximize benefits), practitioner nonmaleficence (minimize burdens), and public justice (ensure fairness) are all upheld.

Conclusion

Collaboration with healthcare teams and building trust with stakeholders are fundamental to the success of ethics consultations. By fostering strong relationships, navigating interprofessional dynamics effectively, and being responsive to the needs of all involved, ethics consultants can ensure that ethical considerations are fully integrated into patient care. This approach not only aligns with the Bioethics Program's mission and vision but also enhances the quality and compassion of patient care, promoting a culture of ethical awareness and integrity within healthcare institutions.

***

The following forms, templates, and checklists will support ethics consultants in developing the essential communication, analytical, cultural, and collaboration skills needed to navigate complex ethical issues effectively. They provide practical, structured approaches that align with the needs of an interprofessional team and ensure that the ethics consultation process is thorough, culturally sensitive, and collaborative.

***

3.1 Active Listening and Empathy Checklist

Purpose: To guide ethics consultants in practicing active listening and empathy during consultations, ensuring that all stakeholders feel heard and understood.

Before the Conversation

- ☐ Prepare by reviewing relevant case details.
- ☐ Set aside personal biases and preconceived notions.
- ☐ Create a calm, private environment for the discussion.

During the Conversation

- ☐ Maintain eye contact and open body language.
- ☐ Allow the speaker to express their thoughts without interruption.
- ☐ Reflect back what you've heard to confirm understanding.
- ☐ Ask open-ended questions to encourage further sharing.
- ☐ Validate the speaker's emotions and perspectives.
- ☐ Offer supportive responses that demonstrate empathy.

After the Conversation

- ☐ Summarize key points and next steps.
- ☐ Thank the speaker for sharing their thoughts and feelings.
- ☐ Reflect on the conversation to identify any areas for improvement in active listening or empathy.

Consultant Name: ______________________________

Date/Time Completed: ______________________________

***

3.2 Facilitating Difficult Conversations Template

Purpose: To provide a structured approach to managing difficult conversations in ethics consultations, ensuring a respectful and constructive dialogue.

Preparation

- ☐ Identify the key issues and emotions involved in the conversation.
- ☐ Set clear goals for the conversation (e.g., resolving a conflict, making a decision).
- ☐ Plan how to introduce the conversation and set the tone.

Introduction

- **Start with Respect**: Begin by acknowledging the difficulty of the conversation and expressing respect for all parties involved.
- **Set Ground Rules**: Establish rules for respectful communication, such as no interruptions and maintaining confidentiality.

Facilitation

- **Encourage Open Dialogue**: Invite each participant to share their perspective and feelings.
- **Manage Emotions**: Acknowledge and address heightened emotions, using de-escalation techniques if necessary.
- **Reframe Negative Statements**: Help participants see issues from different perspectives by reframing negative or accusatory statements in a more positive light.
- **Seek Common Ground**: Identify areas of agreement that can serve as a foundation for resolving the issue.
- **Guide Towards Solutions**: Facilitate a discussion on possible solutions, ensuring that all voices are heard and considered.

Conclusion

- **Summarize Agreements**: Recap the key points of agreement and any decisions made.
- **Plan Next Steps**: Outline the next steps and responsibilities for all parties.
- **Thank Participants**: Acknowledge the effort and openness of all participants.

Consultant Name: ______________________________________

Date/Time Completed: __________________________________

***

3.3 Conflict Resolution and Mediation Checklist

Purpose: To guide ethics consultants through the process of mediating conflicts and resolving disputes among patients, families, and healthcare providers.

Identify the Conflict

- ☐ Clarify the nature of the conflict and the parties involved.
- ☐ Gather information about the underlying causes and perspectives of each party.
- ☐ Determine if there are any immediate safety or care concerns.

Plan the Mediation

- ☐ Schedule a meeting with all relevant parties.
- ☐ Choose a neutral, private location for the mediation.
- ☐ Set the agenda and objectives for the mediation session.

During the Mediation

- **Establish Ground Rules**: Begin by setting rules for respectful communication and confidentiality.
- **Facilitate Open Communication**: Allow each party to express their views and feelings without interruption.
- **Identify Common Interests**: Highlight areas where the parties' interests align.
- **Explore Possible Solutions**: Encourage brainstorming of potential solutions that are acceptable to all parties.
- **Negotiate a Resolution**: Guide the parties towards a mutually agreeable resolution, ensuring that ethical principles are upheld.

After the Mediation

- ☐ Document the agreed-upon resolution and any action items.

- ☐ Follow up with the parties to ensure the resolution is implemented.
- ☐ Reflect on the mediation process and identify areas for improvement.

Consultant Name: ______________________________
Date/Time Completed: ______________________________

***

3.4 Systematic Ethical Analysis Worksheet

Purpose: To help ethics consultants systematically analyze ethical dilemmas using a structured approach, ensuring comprehensive consideration of all relevant factors.

Step 1: Identify the Ethical Dilemma

- ☐ What is the primary ethical issue or conflict?
- ☐ Who are the stakeholders involved?
- ☐ What are the relevant facts and circumstances?

Step 2: Gather Relevant Information

- ☐ Medical facts (diagnosis, prognosis, treatment options).
- ☐ Patient's preferences, values, and goals.
- ☐ Legal and institutional policies.
- ☐ Cultural and religious considerations.
- ☐ Input from family members and healthcare providers.

Step 3: Apply Ethical Principles

- **Patient Autonomy** (Informed Consent): How does the patient's autonomy factor into this dilemma?
- **Practitioner Beneficence** (Maximize Benefits): What actions are in the patient's best interest?
- **Practititoner Nonmaleficence** (Minimize Burdens): How can harm be minimized or avoided?
- **Public Justice** (Ensure Fairness): Are there fairness or equity considerations?

Step 4: Explore Ethical Theories and Frameworks

- ☐ Which ethical theories (e.g., virtue, deontology, utilitarianism) are relevant?
- ☐ How do these theories guide decision-making in this case?

Step 5: Develop and Evaluate Options

- ☐ List possible courses of action.
- ☐ Evaluate the ethical implications of each option.
- ☐ Consider the potential consequences for all stakeholders.

Step 6: Make a Recommendation

- ☐ What is the recommended course of action?
- ☐ How does this recommendation align with ethical principles and the patient's values?
- ☐ Are there any contingencies or follow-up actions required?

Consultant Name: ___________________________________

Date/Time Completed: _________________________________

***

3.5 Cultural Competence Consultation Guide

Purpose: To ensure that ethics consultants approach each consultation with cultural competence and sensitivity, respecting diverse values and beliefs.

Pre-Consultation Preparation

- ☐ Identify the cultural backgrounds of the patient and family members.
- ☐ Research relevant cultural norms, values, and healthcare practices.
- ☐ Be aware of your own cultural biases and assumptions.

During the Consultation

- ☐ Use culturally appropriate communication styles (e.g., language, non-verbal cues).
- ☐ Involve cultural mediators or interpreters if necessary.
- ☐ Respect religious and cultural beliefs that influence healthcare decisions.
- ☐ Acknowledge and address any cultural misunderstandings or conflicts.

Incorporating Cultural Values into Ethical Analysis

- ☐ How do the patient's cultural beliefs and values influence their healthcare decisions?
- ☐ Are there cultural practices that should be respected and incorporated into the care plan?
- ☐ How can ethical principles be applied in a way that honors the patient's cultural context?

Post-Consultation Reflection

- [ ] Reflect on the consultation process and the role of cultural competence.
- [ ] Identify any areas where cultural sensitivity could be improved.
- [ ] Plan for future consultations with similar cultural considerations.

Consultant Name: ______________________________

Date/Time Completed: ______________________________

***

3.6 Interprofessional Collaboration Checklist

Purpose: To guide ethics consultants in effectively collaborating with interprofessional healthcare teams, ensuring integrated and comprehensive ethical decision-making.

Building Relationships

- ☐ Identify key members of the healthcare team.
- ☐ Understand the roles and perspectives of each team member.
- ☐ Establish open lines of communication and regular meetings.

Facilitating Collaboration

- ☐ Encourage input from all team members during consultations.
- ☐ Address any power dynamics or conflicts within the team.
- ☐ Promote mutual respect and understanding among team members.

Integrating Ethical Recommendations

- ☐ Ensure that ethical recommendations are communicated clearly to all team members.
- ☐ Collaborate with the team to integrate recommendations into the patient's care plan.
- ☐ Monitor the implementation of recommendations and provide support as needed.

Reflecting on Team Dynamics

- ☐ Assess the effectiveness of interprofessional collaboration during the consultation.
- ☐ Identify any barriers to effective teamwork and address them proactively.
- ☐ Plan for continuous improvement in interprofessional collaboration.

Consultant Name: ____

Date/Time Completed: ____________________________________

***

Review Questions

True/False Questions:

1. Active listening involves giving full attention to the speaker and acknowledging their feelings.
True or False?

2. Ethics consultants need not consider cultural differences when providing ethics consultation.
True or False?

3. Conflict resolution involves finding mutually acceptable solutions and promoting collaborative decision-making.
True or False?

4. Applying ethical theories and principles to real-world situations is not necessary for ethics consultants.
True or False?

5. Building trust and rapport with stakeholders is essential for successful ethics consultation.
True or False?

Multiple-Choice Questions:

6. Which skill is crucial for ethics consultants to build trust and rapport with stakeholders?
a) Active listening
b) Speed reading
c) Technical writing
d) Public speaking

7. What is one strategy for culturally sensitive consultations?
a) Ignoring cultural differences
b) Using culturally appropriate communication styles
c) Enforcing the consultant's own cultural views
d) Avoiding discussions about culture

Clinical Vignettes:

8. **Scenario:** Mr. Johnson, a patient from a different cultural background, is uncomfortable with the proposed treatment plan because it conflicts with his cultural beliefs. The healthcare team is unsure how to proceed. What is the best course of action?
a) Proceed with the treatment plan regardless of his beliefs
b) Dismiss his concerns as irrelevant
c) Involve an ethics consultant to mediate and ensure cultural sensitivity
d) Transfer the patient to another facility

9. **Scenario:** A conflict arises between the family of a terminally ill patient and the healthcare team regarding the continuation of life-sustaining treatment. The family wants to continue, but the healthcare team believes it is not in the patient's best interest. What is the best course of action?
a) Follow the healthcare team's recommendation without discussion
b) Follow the family's wishes without question
c) Call an ethics consultant to mediate and facilitate a collaborative decision
d) Ignore the conflict and proceed with the healthcare team's plan

10. **Scenario:** Dr. Nguyen is facing an ethical dilemma where a patient requests not to disclose their terminal diagnosis to their family. Dr. Nguyen is unsure how to balance the patient's autonomy with the family's desire/right to know. What is the best course of action?
a) Disclose the diagnosis to the family without informing the patient
b) Respect the patient's wishes and keep the diagnosis confidential
c) Consult with an ethics consultant to analyze the ethical implications and provide guidance
d) Tell the family only partial information

Correct Answers:

1. True
2. False (Ethics consultants must consider cultural differences when providing ethics consultation to ensure that their recommendations are culturally sensitive and respectful of the values and beliefs of the patients and families involved.)
3. True
4. False (Applying ethical theories and principles to real-world situations is essential for ethics consultants. It allows them to analyze ethical dilemmas effectively and provide sound recommendations that are both ethically and legally defensible.)
5. True
6. a) Active listening
7. b) Using culturally appropriate communication styles
8. c) Involve an ethics consultant to mediate and ensure cultural sensitivity
9. c) Call an ethics consultant to mediate and facilitate a collaborative decision
10. c) Consult with an ethics consultant to analyze the ethical implications and provide guidance

***

Further Readings and References

- Aulisio, M. P., Arnold, R. M., & Youngner, S. J. (2000). "*Health Care Ethics Consultation: Nature, Goals, and Competencies.*" In J. Sugarman & D. P. Sulmasy (Eds.), Methods in Medical Ethics (pp. 180-196). Georgetown University Press.
  - *A comprehensive overview discussing the nature and goals of healthcare ethics consultation, with a focus on the competencies required for effective practice.*
- Beauchamp, T. L., & Childress, J. F. (2019). Principles of Biomedical Ethics (8th ed.). Oxford University Press.
  - *This foundational text provides an in-depth discussion of the four principles of biomedical ethics: autonomy, beneficence, nonmaleficence, and justice.*
- American Society for Bioethics and Humanities (ASBH). (2011). Core Competencies for Healthcare Ethics Consultation. ASBH.
  - *This document outlines the essential skills and knowledge required for healthcare ethics consultants, emphasizing the role of ethics consultation in clinical practice.*
- Fiester, A. (2007). "*Mediation and Moral Aporia in the Clinical Setting.*" *The American Journal of Bioethics*, 7(2), 23-25.
  - *An article exploring the role of mediation in clinical ethics consultation, highlighting the importance of conflict resolution and moral reflection.*
- Fisher, R., Ury, W., & Patton, B. (2011). Getting to Yes: Negotiating Agreement Without Giving In (3rd ed.). Penguin Books.
  - *A classic guide on negotiation and conflict resolution, offering practical strategies for finding mutually acceptable solutions.*

- Campinha-Bacote, J. (2002). "The Process of Cultural Competence in the Delivery of Healthcare Services: A Model of Care." Journal of Transcultural Nursing, 13(3), 181-184.
  - *This article introduces a model for cultural competence in healthcare, emphasizing the importance of understanding and respecting cultural differences.*
- Schyve, P. M. (2007). "*Language Differences as a Barrier to Quality and Safety in Health Care: The Joint Commission Perspective." Journal of General Internal Medicine*, 22(Suppl 2), 360-361.
  - *An article discussing the impact of language and cultural differences on healthcare quality and safety, relevant to the practice of culturally sensitive consultations.*
- Halpern, J. (2001). From Detached Concern to Empathy: Humanizing Medical Practice. Oxford University Press.
  - *A book exploring the role of empathy in medical practice, highlighting its importance for building trust and rapport with patients.*
- Nolan, P., & Mockler, D. (2000). "A Comparison of Methods Used to Assess the Communication Skills of Medical Undergraduates." Medical Education, 34(9), 711-715.
  - *This study compares different methods for assessing communication skills in medical education, relevant to the development of active listening and empathy skills in ethics consultants.*
- Zoloth, L. (2002). Health Care and the Ethics of Encounter: A Jewish Discussion of Social Justice. University of North Carolina Press.
  - *A discussion of social justice in healthcare from a Jewish ethical perspective, relevant to the principle of justice in bioethics.*

***

Part IV: Special Topics in Medical Ethics

End-of-Life Decision-Making

Advance Directives and Living Wills

Advance directives and living wills are critical tools that enable individuals to express their wishes regarding medical treatment should they become unable to communicate. Ethics consultants play a pivotal role in ensuring that these directives are respected and integrated into patient care plans, aligning with the principles of patient autonomy (informed consent), practitioner beneficence (maximize benefits), practitioner nonmaleficence (minimize burdens), and public justice (ensure fairness).

- **Patient Autonomy** (Informed Consent): Ethics consultants should facilitate discussions about advance care planning, ensuring that patients or their surrogates understand their diagnosis, prognosis, and the available treatment options. This includes understanding the purpose of each option and the associated benefits and risks. By doing so, ethics consultants support informed consent, allowing patients to make decisions that reflect their reasonable goals, values, and priorities.
- **Practitioner Beneficence** (Maximize Benefits): In honoring advance directives, ethics consultants advocate for actions that enhance the patient's well-being. This involves ensuring that the care provided aligns with the patient's wishes, thereby promoting good outcomes and respecting the patient's goals, values, and priorities.
- **Practitioner Nonmaleficence** (Minimize Burdens): Ethics consultants help prevent harm by ensuring that advance directives are followed, thus avoiding unnecessary or

unwanted interventions. This aligns with the commitment to minimize harm while respecting patient informed consent and the ethical duty to avoid harm.

- **Public Justice** (Ensure Fairness): Advance directives and living wills help ensure that all patients receive fair and equitable treatment, respecting their individual rights and preferences. Ethics consultants must ensure that these directives comply with legal and institutional requirements, upholding the principles of fairness and justice.

Palliative Care and Hospice

Palliative care and hospice services focus on providing comfort and support to patients with serious illnesses. The ethical considerations in these settings often revolve around balancing symptom management, quality of life, and patient autonomy. Ethics consultants are essential in navigating these complex decisions, ensuring that patient preferences are honored and that care is compassionate and respectful.

- **Patient Autonomy** (Informed Consent): Ethics consultants should ensure that patients or surrogates understand the nature of palliative and hospice care, the available options, and the expected outcomes. This understanding supports informed consent, allowing patients to choose care that aligns with their reasonable goals, values, and priorities.
- **Practitioner` Beneficence** (Maximize Benefits): Palliative care and hospice services are inherently focused on enhancing the patient's well-being by managing symptoms and improving quality of life. Ethics consultants advocate for care plans that are compassionate and in line with the patient's wishes, promoting beneficence.
- **Practitioner Nonmaleficence** (Minimize Burdens): In palliative care and hospice settings, ethics consultants help prevent harm by advocating against unnecessary or overly aggressive treatments that do not align with the patient's

goals. This commitment to nonmaleficence ensures that care is appropriate and does not cause unnecessary suffering.

- **Public Justice** (Ensure Fairness): Ensuring equitable access to palliative care and hospice services is essential. Ethics consultants must advocate for fair treatment of all patients, ensuring that care decisions are made transparently and that all patients have access to the support they need.

Ethical Issues in Life-Sustaining Treatments

Life-sustaining treatments, such as mechanical ventilation (MV) and medical nutrition and hydration (MNH), present complex ethical considerations. Decisions about initiating, continuing, or withdrawing these treatments require careful balancing of ethical principles.

- **Patient Autonomy** (Informed Consent): Ethics consultants must ensure that patients or surrogates are fully informed about the implications of life-sustaining treatments, including the benefits, risks, and possible outcomes. Respecting patient autonomy means honoring the patient's preferences and ensuring that consent is informed and voluntary.
- **Practitioner Beneficence** (Maximize Benefits): When considering life-sustaining treatments, ethics consultants should advocate for actions that enhance the patient's well-being. This involves assessing whether the continuation of such treatments aligns with the patient's goals and provides a net benefit.
- **Practitioner Nonmaleficence** (Minimize Burdens): Avoiding harm is a critical consideration in decisions about life-sustaining treatments. Ethics consultants should guide discussions to ensure that treatments do not prolong suffering unnecessarily and that the patient's quality of life is prioritized.
- **Public Justice** (Ensure Fairness): Decisions about life-sustaining treatments should be made fairly and equitably,

with consideration for the broader implications for society. Ethics consultants must ensure that these decisions comply with institutional policies, legal mandates, and medical standards of care, upholding the principle of justice.

Conclusion

Navigating end-of-life decision-making requires a deep commitment to the core bioethical principles of patient autonomy (informed consent), practitioner beneficence (maximize benefits), practitioner nonmaleficence (minimize burdens), and public justice (ensure fairness). Ethics consultants play a crucial role in facilitating discussions, guiding ethical decision-making, and ensuring that patients' wishes are respected. By aligning these decisions with the Bioethics Program's mission and vision, ethics consultants help provide compassionate, respectful, and ethically sound care that honors the dignity and values of each patient.

***

Informed Consent and Capacity

Elements of Informed Consent

Informed consent is a foundational ethical and legal requirement in healthcare, emphasizing respect for patient autonomy. It involves providing patients with comprehensive information about their medical condition, treatment options, associated risks, benefits, and alternatives. Ensuring that patients understand this information and voluntarily agree to the proposed care is essential. Ethics consultants play a crucial role in facilitating this process, ensuring that it aligns with the core bioethical principles and complies with institutional policies and legal mandates.

- **Patient Autonomy** (Informed Consent): Ethics consultants help ensure that patients or their surrogates clearly understand their diagnosis and prognosis, the available treatment options (including the option of no treatment), and the purpose, benefits, and risks associated with each option. This comprehensive understanding supports informed consent, enabling patients to make decisions that align with their reasonable goals, values, and priorities.
- **Practitioner Beneficence** (Maximize Benefits): By advocating for a thorough and respectful informed consent process, ethics consultants contribute to maximizing the patient's well-being. Ensuring that patients are well-informed helps them make choices that enhance their quality of life and align with their health goals.
- **Practitioner Nonmaleficence** (Minimize Burdens): A robust informed consent process minimizes the risk of harm by ensuring that patients are fully aware of potential risks and are making informed decisions. Ethics consultants help prevent harm by ensuring that patients' choices are respected and that

any interventions are aligned with the patient's informed preferences.

- **Public Justice** (Ensure Fairness): Informed consent ensures that all patients receive fair and equitable treatment. Ethics consultants advocate for a standardized and respectful consent process that is accessible to all patients, regardless of background, thereby ensure fairness and justice.

Assessing Decisional Capacity

Assessing a patient's decisional capacity is crucial in situations where their ability to make informed decisions may be impaired. This assessment is a clinical judgment that should be guided by ethical considerations to respect patient autonomy while ensuring their safety and well-being. Ethics consultants can provide valuable insights into these assessments, ensuring that the process aligns with ethical principles.

- **Patient Autonomy** (Informed Consent): Ethics consultants ensure that patients with the capacity to make decisions are respected and that their choices are honored. When capacity is in question, consultants advocate for assessments that accurately reflect the patient's ability to understand, appreciate, and reason about their treatment options and the consequences of their decisions.
- **Practitioner Beneficence** (Maximize Benefits): Ethics consultants guide healthcare providers in conducting capacity assessments that are in the best interest of the patient. By ensuring that assessments are thorough and ethically sound, consultants help support decisions that promote the patient's well-being.
- **Practitioner Nonmaleficence** (Minimize Burdens): Properly assessing decisional capacity helps avoid unnecessary harm. Ethics consultants ensure that assessments are conducted ethically, avoiding coercion or undue influence, and that decisions are made to protect the patient from harm.

- **Public Justice (Ensure Fairness):** Ensuring that capacity assessments are conducted fairly and without bias supports the principle of justice. Ethics consultants advocate for the use of standardized assessment tools and procedures that ensure consistency and fairness in evaluating patients' decision-making abilities.

Addressing Refusal of Treatment

Patients have the right to refuse treatment, even if it may lead to adverse outcomes or death. Navigating these situations requires a careful balance of respecting patient autonomy with the principles of beneficence and nonmaleficence. Ethics consultants provide critical support in these cases, helping to communicate effectively with patients and families and ensuring that decisions are made ethically and compassionately.

- **Patient Autonomy** (Informed Consent): Ethics consultants uphold the right of patients to refuse treatment, provided they have the capacity to make such decisions and are fully informed. Consultants ensure that patients or their surrogates understand the consequences of refusal and that their decisions are respected.
- **Practitioner Beneficence** (Maximize Benefits): While respecting autonomy, ethics consultants also advocate for care plans that offer the best possible outcomes. They work to find a balance that honors the patient's wishes while considering alternative options that could enhance the patient's well-being.
- **Practitioner Nonmaleficence** (Minimize Burdens): Ethics consultants help avoid harm by ensuring that the patient's refusal of treatment is respected when it aligns with the patient's informed and voluntary decision. They help navigate the ethical implications of refusal, ensuring that the decision-making process does not lead to unnecessary suffering or harm.

- **Public Justice** (Ensure Fairness): Ethics consultants advocate for fair and transparent processes when addressing treatment refusal. They ensure that the rights of all patients to accept or refuse treatment are upheld consistently, supporting equity and fairness in healthcare.

Conclusion

Informed consent and the assessment of decisional capacity are critical components of ethical patient care. By emphasizing patient autonomy, ensuring beneficence, minimizing harm, and ensure fairness, ethics consultants play a vital role in guiding these processes. This alignment with the Bioethics Program's mission and vision fosters a healthcare environment where ethical considerations are integral to patient care, enhancing the quality and compassion of medical practice.

***

Confidentiality and Privacy

Legal and Ethical Aspects of Confidentiality

Confidentiality is a core ethical obligation in healthcare, ensuring that patient information is protected and shared only with authorized individuals. It upholds the principle of patient autonomy by respecting patients' privacy and control over their personal information. Ethics consultants play a vital role in guiding healthcare providers on the legal and ethical aspects of confidentiality, helping them navigate complex situations where confidentiality may be challenged.

- **Patient Autonomy** (Informed Consent): Respecting patient confidentiality aligns with the principle of patient autonomy, as it allows patients to have control over who has access to their personal health information. Ethics consultants help ensure that confidentiality practices are transparent and that patients are informed about how their information will be used, thereby supporting informed consent.
- **Practitioner Beneficence** (Maximize Benefits): By maintaining confidentiality, healthcare providers can build trust with patients, which is essential for effective care. Ethics consultants advocate for practices that protect patient information, fostering an environment where patients feel safe to share sensitive information, which can enhance their care and well-being.
- **Practitioner Nonmaleficence** (Minimize Burdens): Protecting patient confidentiality prevents potential harm that could arise from unauthorized disclosure of sensitive information. Ethics consultants provide guidance to healthcare providers on handling patient information securely, thereby minimizing risks and minimize burdens to patients.

- **Public Justice** (Ensure Fairness): Ensuring confidentiality respects the fairness and rights of all patients. Ethics consultants help create policies and procedures that uphold confidentiality, ensuring that all patients are treated equitably and that their privacy rights are consistently protected across the healthcare system.

Managing Sensitive Information

Handling sensitive information requires careful consideration of ethical principles and legal requirements. Ethics consultants assist healthcare providers in managing sensitive information, ensuring that patient privacy is respected and protected. This involves developing and implementing robust policies and procedures for handling sensitive information and providing ongoing training on confidentiality and privacy issues.

- **Patient Autonomy** (Informed Consent): By advocating for clear policies on managing sensitive information, ethics consultants support the patient's right to privacy and autonomy. They ensure that patients are informed about how their data is handled and that their preferences regarding information sharing are respected.
- **Practitioner Beneficence** (Maximize Benefits): Managing sensitive information appropriately ensures that patients' well-being is prioritized. Ethics consultants guide the development of protocols that protect patient information, which in turn helps maintain trust and promotes the patient's overall well-being.
- **Practitioner Nonmaleficence** (Minimize Burdens): Ethics consultants emphasize the importance of protecting sensitive information to prevent potential psychological, social, or financial harm. They advocate for secure data handling practices to avoid unauthorized access or breaches that could negatively impact patients.

- **Public Justice** (Ensure Fairness): Ensuring that sensitive information is managed properly upholds the principle of fairness. Ethics consultants work to establish and maintain policies that ensure all patients' information is handled with the same level of care and respect, promoting justice and equity in healthcare.

Ethical Issues in Electronic Health Records (EHR)

The use of electronic health records (EHR) introduces new ethical challenges related to privacy and confidentiality. Ethics consultants help address these challenges by ensuring that EHR systems are used in ways that protect patient information and uphold ethical standards. They provide guidance on issues such as access controls, data security, and the appropriate use of patient information in EHR systems.

- **Patient Autonomy** (Informed Consent): Ethics consultants advocate for EHR practices that respect patient autonomy by allowing patients to understand and control who has access to their information. They promote transparency in how patient data is used and ensure that patients have opportunities to consent to or restrict access to their information.
- **Practitioner Beneficence** (Maximize Benefits): By ensuring that EHR systems are secure and that access is controlled, ethics consultants help enhance the quality of patient care. They advocate for EHR practices that support comprehensive, well-coordinated care, which ultimately benefits the patient.
- **Practitioner Nonmaleficence** (Minimize Burdens): Ethics consultants play a key role in identifying potential risks associated with EHR systems and advocating for measures to prevent harm. This includes ensuring that data security measures are in place and that only authorized personnel have access to sensitive patient information.
- **Public Justice** (Ensure Fairness): Ethics consultants work to ensure that EHR systems are used fairly and equitably,

supporting the principle of public justice. They advocate for consistent application of privacy standards across all patients, ensuring that no individual's privacy rights are compromised.

Conclusion

Confidentiality and privacy are fundamental to ethical patient care and the protection of patient autonomy. Ethics consultants provide essential guidance to healthcare providers, ensuring that patient information is handled with respect and in compliance with ethical standards and legal requirements. By aligning confidentiality practices with the Bioethics Program's mission and vision, healthcare institutions can foster a culture of trust, fairness, and ethical responsibility, ultimately enhancing the quality and integrity of patient care.

***

Resource Allocation and Justice

Ethical Considerations in Resource Allocation

Resource allocation in healthcare involves making critical decisions about how limited resources are distributed among patients and services. Ethics consultants play a vital role in guiding these decisions, ensuring they align with the principles of patient autonomy (informed consent), practitioner beneficence (maximize benefits), practitioner nonmaleficence (minimize burdens), and public justice (ensure fairness). Ethical resource allocation requires balancing individual patient needs with the broader goal of fairness and equity within the healthcare system.

- **Patient Autonomy** (Informed Consent): Ethics consultants ensure that patients or their surrogates are well-informed about the availability and limitations of healthcare resources. This includes clearly communicating the rationale behind allocation decisions and involving patients in discussions about their care options. By doing so, ethics consultants support the patient's right to make informed decisions based on their reasonable goals, values, and priorities.
- **Practitioner Beneficence** (Maximize Benefits): Ethics consultants advocate for allocation decisions that maximize patient benefits. They work with healthcare providers to develop strategies that prioritize interventions likely to result in the greatest improvement in patient well-being, ensuring that decisions are consistent with the patient's reasonable goals and values, as well as with established medical standards.
- **Practitioner Nonmaleficence** (Minimize Burdens): In resource allocation, ethics consultants emphasize the importance of minimize burdens by ensuring that decisions do

not unduly disadvantage any patient. They guide healthcare providers in identifying and mitigating potential harms associated with resource limitations, ensuring that the principle of nonmaleficence is upheld.

- **Public Justice** (Ensure Fairness): Ensuring fair and equitable distribution of healthcare resources is a fundamental aspect of public justice. Ethics consultants help develop and implement policies that prioritize resource allocation based on ethical criteria, such as medical need, potential benefit, and fairness. They work to ensure that all patients have equitable access to healthcare resources, regardless of their socioeconomic status or other factors.

Rationing Healthcare and Prioritization

Rationing healthcare involves making difficult choices about which patients or treatments to prioritize when resources are limited. Ethics consultants provide essential guidance in navigating these challenging decisions, ensuring that rationing practices are ethical, fair, and transparent.

- **Patient Autonomy** (Informed Consent): Ethics consultants ensure that rationing decisions are communicated transparently to patients and their families. They advocate for patients to be informed about how rationing decisions may affect their care and involve them in discussions about alternative options. This approach supports the principle of informed consent and respects patient autonomy.

- **Practitioner Beneficence** (Maximize Benefits): In guiding rationing decisions, ethics consultants focus on maximizing the benefits to patients. They help establish criteria that prioritize interventions that offer the greatest potential for improving patient health outcomes, ensuring that these decisions are in line with the patient's reasonable goals and values.

- **Practitioner Nonmaleficence** (Minimize Burdens): Ethics consultants work to minimize harm in rationing scenarios by advocating for decisions that avoid unnecessary suffering and adverse outcomes. They encourage healthcare providers to carefully consider the risks associated with rationing and to implement strategies that protect patient safety.
- **Public Justice** (Ensure Fairness): Ethics consultants play a crucial role in ensuring that rationing policies are just and equitable. They work to develop criteria that are fair and consistent, ensuring that all patients are treated equally and that no group is disproportionately affected by resource limitations. This commitment to fairness upholds the principle of public justice.

Addressing Disparities in Healthcare Access

Disparities in healthcare access present significant ethical challenges. Ethics consultants advocate for policies and practices that address these disparities, promoting justice and equity in healthcare.

- **Patient Autonomy** (Informed Consent): Ethics consultants work to ensure that all patients have equal access to information and the opportunity to make informed healthcare decisions. They advocate for patient education initiatives and resources that support informed consent, particularly for underserved populations.
- **Practitioner Beneficence** (Maximize Benefits): Ethics consultants emphasize the importance of providing high-quality care to all patients, regardless of their background or circumstances. They advocate for initiatives that improve access to care and reduce disparities, ensuring that all patients benefit from healthcare advancements.
- **Practitioner Nonmaleficence** (Minimize Burdens): Addressing disparities helps prevent harm that may arise from unequal access to care. Ethics consultants advocate for

policies that reduce barriers to healthcare, such as socioeconomic or geographic factors, thereby minimizing the risk of harm to vulnerable populations.

- **Public Justice** (Ensure Fairness): Promoting equity in healthcare access is a core responsibility of ethics consultants. They work to develop and implement policies that ensure fair treatment for all patients, advocating for systemic changes that address the root causes of disparities and promote justice within the healthcare system.

Conclusion

Ethical considerations in resource allocation, rationing, and addressing healthcare disparities are central to the mission and vision of the Bioethics Program. By integrating the principles of patient autonomy, practitioner beneficence, practitioner nonmaleficence, and public justice, ethics consultants ensure that decisions are made ethically, fairly, and transparently. This alignment fosters an ethical culture that promotes the best interests of patients, enhances the quality and fairness of healthcare, and upholds the integrity of the healthcare system.

***

Research Ethics

Ethical Principles in Clinical Research

Clinical research is foundational to advancing medical knowledge and improving patient care. Ethics consultants are essential in ensuring that research practices adhere to ethical standards, focusing on the protection of research participants and the integrity of the research process. This involves aligning research activities with the principles of patient autonomy (informed consent), practitioner beneficence (maximize benefits), practitioner nonmaleficence (minimize burdens), and public justice (ensure fairness).

- **Patient Autonomy** (Informed Consent): Ethics consultants ensure that research participants are fully informed about the nature of the study, including its purpose, procedures, risks, and benefits. They advocate for clear and comprehensive informed consent processes, allowing participants to make voluntary, well-informed decisions that reflect their reasonable goals, values, and priorities. This process respects and upholds the autonomy of each participant, ensuring that their involvement is based on informed consent.
- **Practitioner Beneficence** (Maximize Benefits): Ethics consultants play a crucial role in ensuring that research designs and interventions aim to maximize benefits for participants. They guide researchers in conducting studies that are likely to lead to improvements in health outcomes, both for the participants involved and for the wider population. This emphasis on beneficence aligns with the commitment to promoting good and enhancing well-being through ethical research practices.

- **Practitioner Nonmaleficence** (Minimize Burdens): Protecting participants from harm is a paramount concern in clinical research. Ethics consultants work closely with researchers to identify and minimize potential risks associated with study participation. They ensure that any risks are justified by the potential benefits and that protective measures are in place to safeguard participants' well-being, thereby upholding the principle of nonmaleficence.
- **Public Justice** (Ensure Fairness): Ethics consultants ensure that the selection of research subjects is fair and equitable, avoiding biases that could lead to the exclusion of specific groups or the exploitation of vulnerable populations. They advocate for research practices that promote justice, ensuring that the benefits and burdens of research are distributed fairly across society. This commitment to public justice supports the ethical conduct of research that benefits all members of the community.

Role of Institutional Review Board (IRB) and Compliance with 45 CFR 46

The oversight of human subjects research is governed by ethical and legal frameworks designed to protect participants' rights and welfare. One of the key components of this oversight is the Institutional Review Board (IRB), as mandated by the *45 Code of Federal Regulations Part 46 (45 CFR 46)*. This regulation codifies the principles of bioethics, including respect for persons, beneficence, and justice, and establishes specific guidelines for the protection of human subjects.

- **Institutional Review Board (IRB) Oversight:** The IRB is a critical body responsible for reviewing and approving research protocols involving human subjects. Its primary function is to ensure that research complies with ethical standards and regulatory requirements. Before any research involving human subjects can begin, it must receive IRB approval, which confirms that the study meets ethical standards for protecting participants.

- **Compliance with 45 CFR 46:** Ethics consultants must ensure that all research involving human subjects is conducted in accordance with 45 CFR 46. This regulation provides a framework for the ethical conduct of research, including requirements for informed consent, risk minimization, and the equitable selection of subjects. Compliance with 45 CFR 46 is not only a legal obligation but also an ethical one, ensuring that research respects and protects the rights and dignity of participants.
- **Informed Consent Requirements:** Under 45 CFR 46, informed consent is a fundamental requirement for all research involving human subjects. Ethics consultants play a pivotal role in ensuring that informed consent processes comply with these regulatory requirements. They help develop consent forms that are clear, comprehensive, and understandable, ensuring that participants are fully informed about the study, including its purpose, risks, benefits, and alternatives.
- **Risk-Benefit Analysis:** The IRB, with the support of ethics consultants, must evaluate the risks and benefits of proposed research. This analysis ensures that the potential benefits justify the risks to participants. Ethics consultants guide researchers in conducting thorough risk assessments and implementing safeguards to protect participants from harm, aligning with the principle of nonmaleficence.
- **Ongoing Monitoring and Reporting:** Compliance with 45 CFR 46 requires ongoing monitoring of research to ensure that ethical standards are maintained throughout the study. Ethics consultants support researchers in establishing monitoring plans and reporting adverse events or changes in research protocols to the IRB. This ongoing oversight is essential to

maintaining the integrity of the research and the safety of participants.

Informed Consent in Research

Informed consent is a cornerstone of ethical research, ensuring that participants understand their involvement and willingly agree to participate. Ethics consultants provide oversight and guidance to ensure that the informed consent process aligns with ethical standards and the principles of the Bioethics Program.

- **Patient Autonomy** (Informed Consent): Ethics consultants advocate for informed consent documents that are clear, comprehensive, and easily understood. They ensure that participants are fully informed about the study, including its purpose, procedures, potential risks, and expected benefits. This process enables participants to make decisions that reflect their reasonable goals, values, and priorities, thereby respecting their autonomy.
- **Practitioner Beneficence** (Maximize Benefits) **and Nonmaleficence** (Minimize Burdens): Ethics consultants guide researchers in balancing the potential benefits of research participation with the need to protect participants from harm. They ensure that informed consent discussions address both the positive outcomes and the risks associated with participation, enabling participants to make well-informed decisions that prioritize their safety and well-being.
- **Public Justice** (Ensure Fairness): Ethics consultants ensure that the informed consent process is accessible and equitable for all potential participants, regardless of their background or circumstances. They advocate for culturally sensitive consent practices that respect the diverse needs and values of research participants, thereby ensure fairness and inclusivity in research.

Addressing Ethical Issues in Experimental Treatments

Experimental treatments, while potentially beneficial, often raise ethical concerns, particularly regarding patient safety and informed consent. Ethics consultants play a key role in navigating these issues, ensuring that experimental treatments are conducted ethically and align with the principles of ppatient autonomy (informed consent), practitioner beneficence (maximize benefits), practitioner nonmaleficence (minimize burdens), and public justice (ensure fairness).

- **Patient Autonomy** (Informed Consent): Ethics consultants emphasize the importance of obtaining informed consent for experimental treatments, ensuring that patients or their surrogates understand the nature of the treatment, its experimental status, potential risks, and expected benefits. This supports patients in making informed choices that align with their reasonable goals, values, and priorities.
- **Practitioner Beneficence** (Maximize Benefits): Ethics consultants work with researchers and healthcare providers to ensure that experimental treatments are designed to maximize potential benefits. They advocate for thorough risk-benefit analyses that support the ethical justification of experimental interventions, prioritizing patient well-being.
- **Practitioner Nonmaleficence** (Minimize Burdens): Ethics consultants help identify and mitigate potential risks associated with experimental treatments. They advocate for monitoring protocols that protect patient safety and ensure that harm is minimized. This commitment to nonmaleficence safeguards patients' rights and well-being throughout the research process.
- **Public Justice** (Ensure Fairness): Ethics consultants ensure that access to experimental treatments is fair and equitable, advocating for criteria that do not discriminate against specific patient groups. They promote transparency in the selection

process and advocate for policies that ensure all patients have the opportunity to participate in experimental treatments, aligning with the principles of fairness and justice.

Conclusion

Ethics consultants are integral to ensuring that clinical research upholds the highest ethical standards, respects patient autonomy, promotes beneficence, avoids harm, and ensures justice. By aligning research practices with these core principles and complying with regulatory requirements such as 45 CFR 46, ethics consultants support the mission and vision of the Bioethics Program, fostering ethical research that respects the dignity of participants and contributes to the advancement of medical knowledge. This approach enhances the integrity of research, ensuring that it is conducted with respect, fairness, and compassion.

***

The following forms, templates, and checklists are designed to help ethics consultants and interprofessional teams navigate complex ethical issues. By providing structured tools for analysis, documentation, and communication, these resources enhance the quality and consistency of ethics consultations, ensuring that decisions are made ethically and with the highest standards of care.

***

4.1 Advance Directives and Living Wills Checklist

Purpose: To guide ethics consultants in discussing and respecting advance directives and living wills, ensuring that patient wishes are honored.

Preparation

- ☐ Review the patient's medical records to identify any existing advance directives or living wills.
- ☐ Confirm the validity and current applicability of the documents.
- ☐ Familiarize yourself with state-specific laws regarding advance directives.

Discussion with Patient/Family

- ☐ Initiate a conversation about the importance of advance directives and living wills.
- ☐ Clarify the patient's goals, values, and priorities related to end-of-life care.
- ☐ Explain the implications of the advance directives in various clinical scenarios.
- ☐ Address any questions or concerns raised by the patient or family.

Integration into Care Plan

- ☐ Ensure that the patient's wishes as outlined in the advance directives are incorporated into the care plan.
- ☐ Communicate the directives to the entire healthcare team.
- ☐ Document all discussions and decisions related to advance directives in the patient's record.

Follow-Up

- ☐ Revisit advance directives periodically, especially if the patient's condition changes.
- ☐ Update documentation as necessary to reflect any changes in the patient's wishes.
- ☐ Provide ongoing support to the patient and family in understanding and implementing advance directives.

Consultant Name: ________________________________

Date/Time Completed: ________________________________

***

4.2 Palliative Care and Hospice Ethics Consultation Template

Purpose: To ensure that ethical issues in palliative care and hospice are addressed comprehensively, respecting patient autonomy and quality of life.

Patient: ______________________________
Diagnosis: ______________________________
Current Treatment Plan: ______________________
Advance Directives:

- ☐ Yes [If Yes, specify]
- ☐ No

Ethical Issues Identified

- ☐ Symptom management vs. quality of life.
- ☐ Patient autonomy in end-of-life decisions.
- ☐ Conflicts between family wishes and patient's preferences.
- ☐ Withholding/withdrawing life-sustaining treatments.
- ☐ Other: ____________________

Stakeholder Engagement

- **Healthcare Team**: (List members involved)
- **Family Members**: (List individuals consulted)
- **Patient**: (If applicable, note patient's involvement in decisions)

Ethical Analysis

- **Autonomy**: How does the patient's autonomy guide decision-making?
- **Beneficence**: What are the best interests of the patient?
- **Nonmaleficence**: How can harm be minimized?
- **Justice**: Are there fairness or equity concerns?

Recommendations

- ☐ Continue current care plan with adjustments:____________
- ☐ Transition to comfort-focused care (palliative care/ hospice).
- ☐ Facilitate a family meeting to discuss care goals.
- ☐ Other: ____

Follow-Up Actions

- ☐ Ensure implementation of care plan changes.
- ☐ Schedule follow-up consultation with the healthcare team.
- ☐ Provide additional resources to the family on end-of-life care.
- ☐ Document all discussions and decisions in the patient's record.

Consultant Name: ___________________________________

Date/Time Completed: ________________________________

***

4.3 Informed Consent and Capacity Assessment Form

Purpose: To assist ethics consultants in evaluating and documenting informed consent and decisional capacity, ensuring patient autonomy is respected.

Patient: ______________________________

Age: ______________________________

Diagnosis: ______________________________

Proposed Treatment/Procedure: ______________________________

Elements of Informed Consent

- ☐ Explanation of the diagnosis and treatment options.
- ☐ Discussion of potential risks and benefits.
- ☐ Alternatives to the proposed treatment.
- ☐ Assessment of the patient's understanding.
- ☐ Confirmation that consent is given voluntarily.

Capacity Assessment

- **Cognitive Function**: (Describe the patient's ability to understand, appreciate, reason, and express a choice.)
- **Emotional State**: (Note any factors that may impair capacity, such as anxiety, depression, or delirium.)
- **Use of Standardized Tools**: (Specify tools used, e.g., Mini-Mental State Examination (MMSE), MacCAT-T.)
- **Assessment Outcome**: [ ] Has capacity [ ] Lacks capacity (If lacks, specify surrogate decision-maker.)

Ethical Considerations

- ☐ Respecting patient autonomy.
- ☐ Balancing beneficence and nonmaleficence.
- ☐ Addressing any conflicts or concerns raised by family or healthcare team.

Consultation Outcome

- ☐ Proceed with the patient's informed consent.
- ☐ Refer to a surrogate decision-maker.
- ☐ Re-evaluate capacity after intervention (e.g., treatment of delirium).
- ☐ Document all discussions and decisions in the patient's record.

Consultant Name: ______________________________

Date/Time Completed: ______________________________

***

4.4 Confidentiality and Privacy Checklist

Purpose: To ensure that patient confidentiality is protected and that sensitive information is managed ethically and legally.

Review of Legal and Ethical Guidelines

- ☐ Familiarize with relevant laws (e.g., HIPAA) and institutional policies on confidentiality.
- ☐ Understand the ethical principles governing patient privacy and confidentiality.

Managing Sensitive Information

- ☐ Identify what constitutes sensitive information in the patient's case.
- ☐ Ensure that sensitive information is accessed only by authorized personnel.
- ☐ Use secure methods for storing and transmitting patient information.

EHR-Specific Considerations

- ☐ Implement access controls to restrict who can view or edit patient records.
- ☐ Regularly audit access logs to monitor for unauthorized access.
- ☐ Provide training on EHR privacy and security practices to all healthcare providers.

Responding to Breaches of Confidentiality

- ☐ Report any breaches immediately according to institutional protocol.
- ☐ Inform the patient and involved parties as required by law.
- ☐ Take corrective actions to prevent future breaches.

Consultation Documentation

- ☐ Document all confidentiality-related discussions and decisions.
- ☐ Ensure that patient privacy is respected in all documentation and communication.

Consultant Name: ________________________________

Date/Time Completed: ________________________________

***

4.5 Resource Allocation and Justice Ethics Consultation Template

Purpose: To guide ethics consultants in addressing ethical issues related to resource allocation and ensuring fair and equitable decisions.

Patient(s): ______________________________________

Resource in Question: ______________________________

Context (e.g., pandemic, shortage): ____________________

Ethical Considerations

- **Justice**: How will resources be allocated fairly?
- **Beneficence**: What is the best use of limited resources to benefit the greatest number?
- **Nonmaleficence**: How can harm be minimized for those who do not receive resources?
- **Autonomy**: How are patient preferences factored into allocation decisions?

Stakeholder Engagement

- **Healthcare Team**: (List members involved)
- **Patients/Families**: (Describe their involvement in the decision-making process)

Analysis and Recommendations

- ☐ Develop criteria for resource allocation (e.g., first come, first served, clinical need).
- ☐ Ensure transparency in the decision-making process.
- ☐ Address any potential disparities in access to resources.
- ☐ Consider the long-term implications of resource allocation decisions.

Follow-Up and Implementation

- ☐ Communicate allocation decisions to all stakeholders.
- ☐ Monitor the impact of allocation decisions on patient outcomes.
- ☐ Review and refine allocation criteria as needed.
- ☐ Document the decision-making process and outcomes in the patient's record.

Consultant Name: ________________________________

Date/Time Completed: ______________________________

***

4.6 Research Ethics Consultation Checklist

Purpose: To guide ethics consultants in evaluating and addressing ethical issues in clinical research, ensuring participant protection and ethical integrity.

Pre-Consultation Review

- ☐ Review the research protocol and informed consent documents.
- ☐ Understand the ethical principles relevant to the research study (e.g., respect for persons, beneficence, justice).

Informed Consent Evaluation

- ☐ Ensure that the informed consent process is comprehensive and understandable.
- ☐ Confirm that participants are fully aware of the risks, benefits, and their rights.
- ☐ Verify that consent is voluntary and free from coercion.

Risk-Benefit Analysis

- ☐ Assess whether the potential benefits of the research outweigh the risks.
- ☐ Consider the fair selection of research subjects and the equitable distribution of risks and benefits.

Ongoing Ethical Oversight

- ☐ Monitor the implementation of the research study to ensure ongoing adherence to ethical standards.
- ☐ Address any ethical concerns that arise during the course of the research.

Post-Consultation Documentation

- ☐ Document the ethical analysis, recommendations, and any decisions made.
- ☐ Ensure that all stakeholders are informed of the consultation outcomes and any follow-up actions.

Consultant Name: ___________________________
Date/Time Completed: ___________________________

***

Review Questions

True/False Questions:

1. Advance directives allow individuals to express their medical treatment wishes if they become unable to communicate.
True or False?

2. Ethics consultants play no role in ensuring that advance directives are respected.
True or False?

3. Life-sustaining treatments always must be continued regardless of the patient's wishes or quality of life.
True or False?

4. Informed consent requires providing patients with adequate information about their treatment options.
True or False?

5. Assessing a patient's decisional capacity is not crucial when their ability to understand and make decisions is in question.
True or False?

Multiple-Choice Questions:

6. Which of the following is a key responsibility of ethics consultants in end-of-life decision-making?
a) Ignoring patient preferences
b) Ensuring that patient preferences are honored
c) Making decisions without consulting the family
d) Focusing solely on legal aspects

7. What is an important element of informed consent?
a) Providing patients with only the benefits of the treatment
b) Ensuring patients voluntarily agree to the proposed care
c) Discussing only the risks of the treatment
d) Making decisions on behalf of the patient

Clinical Vignettes:

8. **Scenario:** Mr. Green, a patient with terminal cancer, has an advance directive requesting no resuscitation. His family insists on continuing aggressive treatment. What is the best course of action?
a) Follow the family's wishes and continue treatment
b) Ignore the advance directive and resuscitate if necessary
c) Involve an ethics consultant to facilitate a discussion respecting Mr. Green's wishes
d) Transfer the patient to another hospital

9. **Scenario:** Mrs. Brown refuses a life-saving surgery due to her personal beliefs. The healthcare team is concerned about her decision. What is the best course of action?
a) Proceed with the surgery without her consent
b) Respect her decision and do not intervene further
c) Involve an ethics consultant to ensure informed consent and explore her decisional capacity
d) Transfer her to another hospital without further discussion

10. **Scenario:** Dr. Williams is treating a patient who has requested an experimental treatment not yet approved. The patient is fully informed about the risks and is desperate for any possible benefit. What is the best course of action?
a) Provide the experimental treatment immediately
b) Deny the request and provide standard care
c) Seek guidance from an ethics consultant to analyze the ethical implications and provide recommendations
d) Refer the patient to another doctor who may provide the treatment

Correct Answers:

1. True
2. False (Ethics consultants play a crucial role in ensuring that advance directives are respected, helping to integrate these directives into patient care plans and ensuring that patients' wishes are honored.)
3. False (Life-sustaining treatments do not always have to be continued regardless of the patient's wishes or quality of life. Ethics consultants help ensure that decisions about continuing or withdrawing life-sustaining treatments align with the patient's wishes and consider the ethical principles of autonomy, beneficence, nonmaleficence, and justice.)
4. True
5. False (Assessing a patient's decisional capacity is crucial when their ability to understand and make decisions is in question. It is essential to ensure that any decisions made are informed, voluntary, and in line with the patient's values and best interests.)
6. b) Ensuring that patient preferences are honored
7. b) Ensuring patients voluntarily agree to the proposed care
8. c) Involve an ethics consultant to facilitate a discussion respecting Mr. Green's wishes
9. c) Involve an ethics consultant to ensure informed consent and explore her decisional capacity
10. c) Seek guidance from an ethics consultant to analyze the ethical implications and provide recommendations

***

Further Readings and References

- Beauchamp, T. L., & Childress, J. F. (2019). Principles of Biomedical Ethics (8th ed.). Oxford University Press.
  - *This foundational text provides an in-depth discussion of the four principles of biomedical ethics: autonomy, beneficence, nonmaleficence, and justice.*
- Quill, T. E., & Cassel, C. K. (1995). "Nonabandonment: A Central Obligation for Physicians." *Annals of Internal Medicine*, 122(5), 368-374.
  - *An article discussing the ethical obligation of nonabandonment in the physician-patient relationship, relevant to the role of ethics consultants in ensuring continuous care.*
- Jonsen, A. R., Siegler, M., & Winslade, W. J. (2015). Clinical Ethics: A Practical Approach to Ethical Decisions in Clinical Medicine (8th ed.). McGraw-Hill Education.
  - *A practical guide addressing ethical dilemmas in clinical practice, with case studies and frameworks for decision-making.*
- Truog, R. D., et al. (2008). "*Recommendations for End-of-Life Care in the Intensive Care Unit: A Consensus Statement by the American College of Critical Care Medicine." Critical Care Medicine*, 36(3), 953-963.
  - *Consensus recommendations on end-of-life care in the ICU, highlighting the ethical considerations and the role of ethics consultation in decision-making.*
- Campbell, M. L., & Guzman, J. A. (2003). "*Impact of a Proactive Approach to Improve End-of-Life Care in a Medical ICU." Chest*, 123(1), 266-271.
  - *This article explores the impact of proactive end-of-life care planning in intensive care settings, relevant to discussions on advance directives and living wills.*

- Grady, C. (2010). "*Do IRBs Protect Human Research Participants?*" *JAMA*, 304(10), 1122-1123.
  - *This article discusses the role of Institutional Review Boards (IRBs) in protecting human research participants, relevant to the ethics consultation process in research settings.*
- Dubler, N. N., & Liebman, C. B. (2011). Bioethics Mediation: A Guide to Shaping Shared Solutions. Vanderbilt University Press.
  - *A guide on using mediation techniques in bioethics consultations to shape shared solutions and resolve conflicts.*
- Fisher, R., Ury, W., & Patton, B. (2011). Getting to Yes: Negotiating Agreement Without Giving In (3rd ed.). Penguin Books.
  - *A classic guide on negotiation and conflict resolution, offering practical strategies for finding mutually acceptable solutions.*
- Campinha-Bacote, J. (2002). "*The Process of Cultural Competence in the Delivery of Healthcare Services: A Model of Care.*" *Journal of Transcultural Nursing*, 13(3), 181-184.
  - *This article introduces a model for cultural competence in healthcare, emphasizing the importance of understanding and respecting cultural differences.*
- Post, S. G., Blustein, J., Gordon, E. J., & Mishkin, D. (Eds.). (2007). Handbook for Health Care Ethics Committees. Johns Hopkins University Press.
  - *A practical guide for ethics committees, with chapters on conducting ethics consultations, policy development, and ethics education.*
- Fins, J. J., & Bacchetta, M. D. (1995). "*Framing the Clinical Ethics Case Consultation: A Pedagogical and Problem-Oriented Approach.*" *Journal of Clinical Ethics*, 6(3), 239-251.
  - *This article offers a pedagogical approach to conducting ethics consultations, focusing on case framing and problem-solving strategies.*

- Emanuel, E. J., Wendler, D., & Grady, C. (2000). "*What Makes Clinical Research Ethical?*" *JAMA*, 283(20), 2701-2711.
  - *This article outlines the ethical principles guiding clinical research, including informed consent, risk-benefit analysis, and the fair selection of research subjects.*
- Pellegrino, E. D., & Thomasma, D. C. (1993). The Virtues in Medical Practice. Oxford University Press.
  - *A philosophical exploration of the virtues essential to medical practice, including the role of ethics consultation in promoting virtuous behavior in healthcare.*
- Schyve, P. M. (2007). "*Language Differences as a Barrier to Quality and Safety in Health Care: The Joint Commission Perspective.*" *Journal of General Internal Medicine*, 22(Suppl 2), 360-361.
  - *An article discussing the impact of language and cultural differences on healthcare quality and safety, relevant to the practice of culturally sensitive consultations.*

***

Part V: Education and Professional Development

Ethics Education and Training

Designing Effective Ethics Education Programs

Ethics education is a cornerstone of the Bioethics Program, essential for preparing healthcare providers and ethics consultants to address complex ethical dilemmas. To align with the mission of maximizing the patient's best interests and ensuring informed, ethical decision-making, ethics education programs must be well-designed, relevant, and impactful. These programs should incorporate the four core bioethical principles—patient autonomy (informed consent), practitioner beneficence (maximize benefits), practitioner nonmaleficence (minimize burdens), and public justice (ensure fairness)—and ensure compliance with institutional policies, established medical standards of care, and legal mandates.

- **Incorporating Patient Autonomy** (Informed Consent): Education programs must emphasize the importance of patient autonomy by teaching healthcare providers how to engage patients and their surrogates in meaningful conversations about their diagnosis, prognosis, and available treatment options. Ethics training should include modules on informed consent, ensuring that providers can effectively communicate the purpose, benefits, and risks of treatment options, and respect patient decisions that reflect their reasonable goals, values, and priorities.
- **Advancing Practitioner Beneficence** (Maximize Benefits): Ethics education should highlight the ethical obligation of healthcare providers to act in the best interest of the patient. Training programs should include case studies and simulations

that demonstrate how to assess and maximize the benefits of proposed interventions. Ethics consultants should be trained to guide healthcare providers in making decisions that promote the patient's well-being, aligning with the principles of beneficence and adhering to medical standards of care and institutional policies.

- **Ensuring Practitioner Nonmaleficence** (Minimize Burdens): Avoiding harm is a fundamental ethical principle that should be integral to ethics education. Programs must equip healthcare providers with the skills to identify potential harms and mitigate risks associated with clinical interventions. Training should include strategies for balancing benefits and harms, emphasizing the importance of adhering to ethical guidelines, institutional policies, and legal requirements to protect patients from unnecessary harm.
- **Advocating for Public Justice** (Ensure Fairness): Ethics education should foster an understanding of fairness and justice in healthcare. Programs must address issues related to equitable access to care, resource allocation, and the broader societal implications of healthcare decisions. By promoting public justice, ethics education ensures that healthcare providers and ethics consultants are prepared to advocate for fair treatment of all patients and to address disparities in healthcare access and outcomes.

Teaching Methods and Tools

To effectively convey these ethical principles, ethics education programs must utilize diverse teaching methods and tools that engage learners and promote ethical reflection.

- **Case Studies and Simulations:** Real-world scenarios can help learners apply ethical principles to complex situations. Ethics consultants should use case studies to illustrate ethical dilemmas and encourage critical thinking. Simulations and role-playing can provide hands-on experience in navigating ethical challenges, enhancing learners' ability to apply ethical principles in clinical practice.

- **Interactive Discussions:** Facilitated discussions encourage active participation and the sharing of diverse perspectives. Ethics consultants should create safe spaces for open dialogue, where learners can discuss ethical issues, share their viewpoints, and learn from others. Interactive discussions foster a deeper understanding of ethical principles and their application in real-life scenarios.
- **Innovative Teaching Approaches:** Ethics education programs should incorporate innovative methods such as digital tools, online platforms, and multimedia resources to enhance learning. Interactive modules, webinars, and virtual reality simulations can make ethics education more engaging and accessible, accommodating different learning styles and needs.

Assessing Learning Outcomes

Evaluating the effectiveness of ethics education programs is critical to ensuring that they achieve their objectives. Ethics consultants should develop robust assessment tools that measure learners' understanding of ethical principles and their ability to apply them in clinical practice.

- **Formative Assessments:** Ongoing assessments during the training process help gauge learners' progress and understanding. Ethics consultants should use quizzes, reflective exercises, and feedback sessions to monitor learning and identify areas where additional support is needed. Formative assessments provide valuable insights into the effectiveness of the education program and guide adjustments to enhance learning.
- **Summative Assessments:** At the conclusion of the training, summative assessments evaluate the overall effectiveness of the ethics education program. These assessments can include

written exams, practical evaluations, and objective structured clinical examinations (OSCEs) to test learners' knowledge, skills, and ethical decision-making abilities. Summative assessments ensure that learners have met the program's learning objectives and are prepared to apply ethical principles in their practice.

- **Feedback Mechanisms:** Gathering feedback from learners is essential for continuous improvement of ethics education programs. Ethics consultants should use surveys, interviews, and focus groups to collect feedback on the program's content, teaching methods, and effectiveness. This feedback informs ongoing program development and ensures that ethics education remains relevant and impactful.

Conclusion

The integration of ethics education into healthcare training is vital for fostering a culture of ethical awareness, understanding, and continuous learning among healthcare providers and ethics consultants. By designing and implementing comprehensive ethics education programs that align with the Bioethics Program's mission and vision, healthcare institutions can ensure that ethical considerations are at the forefront of patient care and decision-making. These programs empower healthcare providers to respect patient autonomy, promote beneficence, avoid harm, and advocate for justice, ultimately enhancing the quality and compassion of healthcare delivery.

***

Professional Growth and Development

Continuing Education and Certification

Continuing education and certification are pivotal for the professional growth of ethics consultants, ensuring they remain knowledgeable and competent in addressing complex ethical dilemmas. These opportunities align with the Bioethics Program's mission to promote ethical awareness and continuous education. Ethics consultants should actively pursue continuing education, such as workshops, conferences, and online courses, and seek certification through recognized professional organizations to enhance their skills in applying the four core bioethical principles—patient autonomy (informed consent), practitioner beneficence (maximize benefits), practitioner nonmaleficence (minimize burdens), and public justice (ensure fairness).

- **Emphasizing Patient Autonomy** (Informed Consent): Continuing education programs should include training on effectively engaging patients and their surrogates in discussions about their healthcare decisions. Ethics consultants must be adept at helping healthcare providers ensure that patients are fully informed about their diagnosis, prognosis, treatment options, and the associated risks and benefits, thereby supporting informed consent and aligning care with the patient's reasonable goals, values, and priorities.
- **Advancing Practitioner Beneficence** (Maximize Benefits): Ethics consultants should engage in educational opportunities that reinforce their commitment to promoting the well-being of patients. Training should focus on enhancing the ability to assess the benefits of proposed treatments and to advocate for care that aligns with the patient's best interests. Ethics consultants must ensure that healthcare providers' actions

promote good outcomes while adhering to medical standards of care, institutional policies, and legal mandates.

- **Ensuring Practitioner Nonmaleficence** (Minimize Burdens): Avoiding harm is a key principle in ethical practice. Ethics consultants must participate in continuing education that focuses on risk assessment and harm reduction strategies. Training should equip consultants with the tools to guide healthcare providers in identifying and mitigating potential risks to patients, ensuring that ethical guidelines are followed, and that unnecessary harm is avoided.
- **Advocating for Public Justice** (Ensure Fairness): Ethics consultants should seek training that addresses issues of fairness and equity in healthcare. Continuing education programs should cover topics such as resource allocation, healthcare disparities, and the societal implications of healthcare decisions. By understanding these issues, ethics consultants can advocate for policies and practices that promote justice and equitable treatment for all patients.

Networking and Professional Organizations

Active engagement in networking and participation in professional organizations provide ethics consultants with valuable opportunities for professional growth and development. These organizations offer resources, support, and a platform for sharing best practices, thereby enhancing the consultant's ability to apply the four core bioethical principles in clinical practice.

- **Connecting with Peers:** Networking with other ethics consultants and healthcare professionals allows for the exchange of knowledge and experiences. These interactions can lead to a deeper understanding of ethical issues and the development of innovative approaches to ethics consultation. Professional organizations often facilitate these connections through conferences, seminars, and online forums.

- **Staying Informed:** Participation in professional organizations keeps ethics consultants updated on the latest developments in bioethics, healthcare policy, and legal mandates. These organizations provide access to research, publications, and training opportunities that are essential for maintaining competence and ensuring that ethical practices are aligned with current standards and guidelines.
- **Professional Advocacy:** Ethics consultants can play a role in shaping the field of bioethics by engaging with professional organizations. Through participation in committees, working groups, and advocacy efforts, consultants can contribute to the development of ethical standards, policies, and educational programs that promote the principles of patient autonomy, practitioner beneficence, practitioner nonmaleficence, and public justice.

Self-Care and Avoiding Burnout

The work of ethics consultants often involves navigating emotionally challenging situations, which can lead to stress and burnout. To maintain their well-being and effectiveness, ethics consultants must prioritize self-care and develop strategies to manage stress. This aligns with the Bioethics Program's commitment to fostering ethical awareness and ensuring the well-being of those involved in patient care.

- **Setting Boundaries:** Ethics consultants should establish clear boundaries to maintain a healthy work-life balance. This includes managing workload, setting limits on availability, and taking time for rest and relaxation. Maintaining boundaries helps prevent burnout and ensures that consultants can provide thoughtful and compassionate ethical guidance.
- **Seeking Support:** Ethics consultants should have access to support systems, including peer support groups, counseling services, and professional mentorship. Engaging with colleagues and mentors can provide emotional support, reduce

feelings of isolation, and offer new perspectives on challenging cases.

- **Developing Self-Care Practices:** Ethics consultants should identify and incorporate self-care practices that help them manage stress and maintain resilience. This may include mindfulness techniques, regular physical activity, hobbies, and time with family and friends. By prioritizing their well-being, ethics consultants can remain effective in their role and continue to provide high-quality ethics consultation.

Conclusion

Professional growth and development are integral to the role of ethics consultants, ensuring they are equipped to address ethical challenges in healthcare with competence and compassion. By pursuing continuing education, engaging with professional organizations, and prioritizing self-care, ethics consultants can uphold the principles of patient autonomy (informed consent), practitioner beneficence (maximize benefits), practitioner nonmaleficence (minimize burdens), and public justice (ensure fairness). These efforts align with the Bioethics Program's mission and vision, promoting ethical awareness, understanding, and continuous education among healthcare practitioners and ethics consultants. This commitment to professional development ultimately enhances the quality and compassion of patient care, fostering a culture of ethical excellence within healthcare institutions.

***

Case Studies and Clinical Vignettes

Real-World Examples of Ethical Dilemmas

Case studies and clinical vignettes are essential tools for illustrating real-world ethical dilemmas in healthcare. These examples provide practical insights into the complexities of ethical decision-making, demonstrating the application of the four core bioethical principles: patient autonomy (informed consent), practitioner beneficence (maximize benefits), practitioner nonmaleficence (minimize burdens), and public justice (ensure fairness). Ethics consultants should use case studies to highlight key ethical issues, showcasing effective approaches to ethical analysis and resolution while ensuring alignment with the Bioethics Program's mission and vision.

- **Emphasizing Patient Autonomy** (Informed Consent): Case studies should include scenarios that emphasize the patient's right to informed consent and decision-making based on their reasonable goals, values, and priorities. These examples should illustrate the importance of patients or their surrogates understanding their diagnosis and prognosis, being informed of all available treatment options, comprehending the purpose of each option, evaluating the potential benefits and risks, and providing logical reasons for their decisions. Scenarios should also highlight the surrogate's role in decision-making when the patient lacks decisional capacity, using substituted judgment based on the patient's known preferences.
- **Advancing Practitioner Beneficence** (Maximize Benefits): Ethics consultants should choose case studies that demonstrate actions aimed at enhancing the patient's well-being, in accordance with the principle of beneficence. These examples should show how healthcare providers can advocate for treatment options that maximize benefits to the patient, as

determined by the patient's reasonable goals, values, and priorities. The case studies should also reflect adherence to medical standards of care, institutional policies, and legal mandates, especially when the patient's preferences are not explicitly known.

- **Ensuring Practitioner Nonmaleficence** (Minimize Burdens): Avoiding harm is a critical aspect of ethical practice. Case studies should include examples where ethics consultants and healthcare providers work to minimize unnecessary harm or risks to the patient. These scenarios should illustrate how to balance the need for treatment with the potential for harm, ensuring that ethical guidelines are followed and that patient safety is prioritized. The importance of assessing and mitigating risks should be a key focus, aligning with the principles of patient autonomy, beneficence, and public justice.
- **Advocating for Public Justice** (Ensure Fairness): Case studies should address issues of fairness and equity in healthcare, demonstrating how ethical decisions can impact broader societal concerns. Examples should include scenarios where resource allocation, access to care, and treatment prioritization are at play. These cases should illustrate how to apply the principle of public justice, ensuring that all patients receive fair and equitable treatment, regardless of their socioeconomic status, background, or other factors. Scenarios should highlight how adherence to institutional policies, medical standards, and legal frameworks supports ethical decision-making.

Analysis and Discussion of Case Studies

Analyzing and discussing case studies is a powerful method for enhancing ethical understanding and critical thinking. Ethics consultants should use these discussions to engage learners in exploring the complexities of ethical dilemmas, encouraging them to reflect on how the four core bioethical principles can be applied in real-life situations.

- **Encouraging Ethical Reflection:** Discussions should focus on identifying the ethical issues present in each case study, exploring the different perspectives of patients, families, and healthcare providers. Participants should be encouraged to consider how patient autonomy, practitioner beneficence, practitioner nonmaleficence, and public justice are addressed in each scenario and to propose solutions that align with these principles.
- **Identifying Lessons Learned:** Case study discussions should aim to identify lessons learned from each scenario, highlighting best practices in ethical decision-making. Ethics consultants should facilitate conversations that explore what was done well, what could have been improved, and how similar situations might be handled in the future. This reflective practice promotes continuous improvement and reinforces the importance of ethical principles in guiding clinical decisions.

Lessons Learned and Best Practices

Case studies provide valuable opportunities to identify lessons learned and best practices in ethical decision-making. Ethics consultants should document these lessons and use them to promote continuous improvement in ethics consultation services.

- **Sharing Best Practices:** Ethics consultants should develop a repository of best practices based on case study analysis. Sharing these practices with colleagues and within the broader healthcare community helps build a culture of ethical excellence, ensuring that ethical considerations are integrated into every aspect of patient care and decision-making. This aligns with the Bioethics Program's vision of fostering an ethical culture throughout the healthcare institution.

- **Promoting Continuous Improvement:** By regularly reviewing and updating case studies and best practices, ethics consultants can ensure that their approach to ethics consultation remains relevant and effective. Continuous improvement efforts should focus on enhancing the quality and compassion of patient care, in alignment with the Bioethics Program's mission to maximize the patient's best interests and uphold the principles of patient autonomy, practitioner beneficence, practitioner nonmaleficence, and public justice.

Conclusion

Incorporating case studies and clinical vignettes into ethics consultation and education provides a practical and impactful way to demonstrate the application of bioethical principles in real-world scenarios. By focusing on patient autonomy (informed consent), practitioner beneficence (maximize benefits), practitioner nonmaleficence (minimize burdens), and public justice (ensure fairness), these examples support the Bioethics Program's mission and vision, promoting ethical awareness, understanding, and continuous education among healthcare practitioners and ethics consultants. Through thoughtful analysis and discussion of case studies, ethics consultants can foster a culture of ethical reflection and improvement, ultimately enhancing the quality and compassion of patient care.

***

The Future of Medical Ethics Consultation

Evolving Challenges and Opportunities in Medical Ethics Consultation

The field of medical ethics consultation is continually evolving to meet the demands of a rapidly changing healthcare landscape. Advances in medical technology, shifts in healthcare policies, and evolving societal values all contribute to new challenges and opportunities for ethics consultants. To navigate these emerging complexities effectively, ethics consultants must be adaptable, forward-thinking, and committed to ongoing education and ethical reflection.

- **Patient Autonomy and Emerging Technologies:** As new medical technologies emerge, ensuring that patients maintain their right to informed consent is crucial. Ethics consultants play a pivotal role in guaranteeing that patients or their surrogates understand the implications of these technologies on their health. This involves educating patients about their diagnosis, prognosis, and available options, including the option to refuse treatment. Ethics consultants must ensure that patients comprehend the purpose, benefits, and risks associated with each technological intervention. This empowers patients to make informed decisions that align with their reasonable goals, values, and priorities, thereby respecting their autonomy.
- **Enhancing Beneficence in Policy Development:** With changing healthcare policies, the principle of beneficence must remain a central consideration. Ethics consultants should advocate for policies that prioritize the patient's best interests, promoting actions that enhance the patient's well-being. This requires a deep understanding of how new policies impact patient care and the ability to guide healthcare providers in

aligning their practices with these policies while staying true to the principle of beneficence. Consultants should help ensure that policy developments support the highest standards of patient care and align with the patients' reasonable goals, values, and priorities.

- **Addressing Nonmaleficence with New Interventions:** As medical practices evolve, ethics consultants must remain vigilant in upholding the principle of nonmaleficence—avoiding unnecessary harm to patients. New medical interventions must be scrutinized to ensure they do not introduce undue risk or harm. Ethics consultants should guide healthcare providers in conducting thorough risk-benefit analyses, ensuring that interventions are not only beneficial but also safe for patients. This includes staying informed about emerging risks and advocating for safeguards that protect patient well-being.
- **Promoting Public Justice in Resource Allocation:** With limited resources and increasing demand, the principle of public justice becomes ever more critical. Ethics consultants should advocate for fair and equitable distribution of healthcare resources, ensuring that all patients have access to necessary care. This includes developing transparent criteria for resource allocation and addressing disparities in access to care. By promoting justice, ethics consultants help uphold the integrity of healthcare institutions and ensure that all patients receive fair treatment, regardless of their background or circumstances.

Final Thoughts on the Role of Ethics Consultants in Healthcare

Ethics consultants are vital to the ethical integrity of healthcare institutions. Their role in ensuring that healthcare practices align with ethical standards and respect patient rights fosters trust, transparency, and moral integrity within the healthcare system. As the field continues to evolve, ethics consultants must remain committed to the principles of patient autonomy (informed consent), practitioner beneficence (maximize benefits), practitioner nonmaleficence (minimize burdens), and public justice (ensure fairness).

- **Commitment to Ethical Reflection and Continuous Improvement:** The dynamic nature of healthcare demands that ethics consultants engage in continuous ethical reflection and improvement. By regularly assessing their practices and adapting to new challenges, ethics consultants ensure that they remain effective advocates for ethical patient care. This commitment to ethical excellence aligns with the Bioethics Program's vision of cultivating a culture of ethical reflection, dialogue, and education throughout the healthcare institution.
- **Enhancing Trust and Transparency:** By providing clear guidance on ethical issues and ensuring that patient rights are respected, ethics consultants build trust between patients, healthcare providers, and institutions. This trust is essential for maintaining open communication and ensuring that patients feel supported in their healthcare journey. Transparency in decision-making processes and ethics consultations further strengthens this trust, contributing to a more ethical and compassionate healthcare environment.

Conclusion

The future of medical ethics consultation is one of ongoing adaptation and commitment to the foundational bioethical principles. By focusing on patient autonomy (informed consent), practitioner beneficence (maximize benefits), practitioner nonmaleficence (minimize burdens), and public justice (ensure fairness), ethics consultants play a critical role in shaping a healthcare system that is both ethically sound and responsive to the needs of patients. Through their dedication to ethical reflection, continuous education, and advocacy for patient rights, ethics consultants help ensure that healthcare institutions remain committed to the highest standards of ethical practice, ultimately enhancing the quality and compassion of patient care.

***

The following templates, forms, and checklists can greatly enhance the efficacy of ethics education, professional development, and case analysis for ethics consultants.

***

5.1 Ethics Education Program Design Template

Purpose: To guide ethics consultants in designing comprehensive and effective ethics education programs for healthcare providers.

Program Title: ____
Target Audience: [ ] Physicians [ ] Nurses [ ] Social Workers
[ ] Administrators [ ] Other: ______________________________

Program Goals:

1.
2.
3.

Learning Objectives:

- By the end of this program, participants will be able to:
  1.
  2.
  3.

Content Outline:

1. Introduction
   - Overview of the program.
   - Importance of ethics in healthcare.
2. Core Ethical Principles
   - Autonomy, Beneficence, Nonmaleficence, Justice.
3. Case Studies and Ethical Dilemmas
   - Real-world examples for discussion.
4. Interactive Sessions
   - Simulations, role-playing exercises.
5. Conclusion and Q&A
   - Summary of key points.
   - Open discussion.

Teaching Methods and Tools:

- ☐ Case Studies
- ☐ Role-Playing
- ☐ Simulations
- ☐ Group Discussions
- ☐ Interactive Polls/Surveys
- ☐ Other:

____

Assessment Methods:

- ☐ Pre- and Post-Program Surveys
- ☐ Knowledge Quizzes
- ☐ Participant Feedback Forms
- ☐ Practical Evaluations (e.g., role-play assessments)
- ☐ Other:

____

Materials and Resources Needed:

- ☐ Handouts
- ☐ PowerPoint Presentations
- ☐ Video Clips
- ☐ Simulation Scenarios
- ☐ Online Learning Platform Access
- ☐ Other:

____

Program Schedule:

- **Session 1**: ______________________ (Date/Time)
- **Session 2**: ______________________ (Date/Time)
- **Session 3**: ______________________ (Date/Time)

Program Evaluation and Follow-Up:

- ☐ Post-Program Survey Distribution
- ☐ Review of Participant Feedback
- ☐ Follow-Up Email with Additional Resources
- ☐ Plan for Continuous Improvement of Program

Program Designer(s): ______________________

Date: ______________________

***

5.2 Professional Development Plan for Ethics Consultants

Purpose: To support the ongoing professional growth of ethics consultants through structured planning and goal-setting.

Consultant Name: ______________________________
Current Role: ______________________________
Date: ______________________________

Professional Development Goals:

- Short-Term Goals (6-12 months):
  1.
  2.
  3.
- Long-Term Goals (1-3 years):
  1.
  2.
  3.

Continuing Education Opportunities:

- ☐ Attend Conferences (List potential conferences): __________
- ☐ Enroll in Online Courses/Webinars (List topics): __________
- ☐ Pursue Certification (Specify certification): ______________
- ☐ Participate in Workshops/Seminars: ____________________
- ☐ Other: ____

Networking and Professional Organizations:

- ☐ Join Professional Organizations (e.g., ASBH, ABPD): ______
- ☐ Attend Networking Events: ____________________________
- ☐ Participate in Online Forums/Communities: ______________
- ☐ Contribute to Professional Publications/Presentations: ______

Self-Care Strategies:

- ☐ Set Boundaries for Work/Life Balance
- ☐ Regularly Engage in Physical Activity
- ☐ Seek Professional Support/Counseling
- ☐ Practice Mindfulness/Relaxation Techniques
- ☐ Schedule Regular Time Off

Mentorship and Peer Support:

- **Mentor Name**: ______________________________________
- Areas of Support:
  - ☐ Career Guidance
  - ☐ Skill Development
  - ☐ Networking Opportunities
  - ☐ Other: ______________________________________
- **Peer Support Group**: (List members and meeting frequency) ______________________________________

Review and Reflection:

- **Progress Review Date**: ______________________________
- **Achievements**: ______________________________________
- Areas for Further Development: __________________________
- **Next Steps**: ____

Consultant Signature: ______________________________

Supervisor/Mentor Signature: ______________________

***

5.3 Case Study Analysis and Reflection Worksheet

Purpose: To guide ethics consultants and learners in analyzing and reflecting on ethical dilemmas presented in case studies.

Case Title: ____
Date: ____
Consultant Name: ____

Summary of the Case:

- Briefly describe the case scenario, including key facts and ethical dilemmas.

Key Ethical Issues Identified:

- List the primary ethical issues raised in the case.

Stakeholder Perspectives:

- **Patient**: ____
- **Family**: ____
- **Healthcare Providers**: ____
- **Ethics Consultant**: ____

Ethical Principles Involved:

- ☐ Patient Autonomy (informed consent)
- ☐ Practitioner Beneficence (maximize benefits)
- ☐ Practitioner Nonmaleficence (minimize burdens)
- ☐ Public Justice (ensure fairness)
- ☐ Other:

____

Ethical Analysis:

- Discuss how each ethical principle applies to the case. Consider conflicting principles and how they were balanced.

Recommendations Provided:

- Detail the recommendations given by the ethics consultant.

Outcome of the Case:

- Describe the resolution of the case and the impact of the ethics consultation.

Lessons Learned:

- Identify key takeaways and best practices from the case.

Personal Reflection:

- Reflect on your own thoughts and feelings about the case. How did it challenge your ethical understanding? What would you do differently in a similar situation?

Future Applications:

- Discuss how the lessons learned from this case can be applied to future ethics consultations.

Follow-Up Actions:

- ☐ Review similar cases or literature for deeper understanding.
- ☐ Discuss the case with a mentor or peer group.
- ☐ Incorporate lessons learned into future practice.

Consultant Signature: ______________________________

***

5.4 Self-Care Checklist for Ethics Consultants

Purpose: To ensure that ethics consultants maintain their well-being and resilience while working in emotionally challenging environments.

Date: ____________________

Consultant Name: ____________________

Work-Life Balance

- ☐ Set clear boundaries between work and personal time.
- ☐ Schedule regular breaks during the workday.
- ☐ Take time off when needed to recharge.

Physical Health

- ☐ Engage in regular physical activity (e.g., walking, yoga, gym).
- ☐ Maintain a balanced diet.
- ☐ Get sufficient sleep (7-8 hours per night).
- ☐ Schedule regular medical check-ups.

Emotional and Mental Well-being

- ☐ Practice mindfulness or relaxation techniques (e.g., meditation, deep breathing).
- ☐ Seek professional counseling or therapy if needed.
- ☐ Stay connected with family and friends for support.
- ☐ Engage in hobbies or activities that bring joy and relaxation.

Professional Support

- ☐ Participate in peer support groups or supervision.
- ☐ Regularly debrief challenging cases with a mentor or colleague.
- ☐ Attend workshops or training on stress management and resilience.

Reflection and Growth

- ☐ Reflect on your experiences and learn from them.
- ☐ Celebrate your successes and acknowledge your challenges.
- ☐ Continuously seek opportunities for personal and professional growth.

Review and Adjust

- ☐ Regularly review and adjust your self-care strategies as needed.
- ☐ Keep track of your well-being and make changes to prevent burnout.

Consultant Signature: ______________________________

***

Review Questions

True/False Questions:

1. Effective ethics education programs should incorporate a range of teaching methods and tools.
True or False?

2. Case studies are not useful in illustrating real-world ethical dilemmas.
True or False?

3. Continuing education and certification are important for the professional growth of ethics consultants.
True or False?

4. Networking and participation in professional organizations provide no real benefit for ethics consultants.
True or False?

5. Self-care is essential for ethics consultants to manage stress and avoid burnout.
True or False?

Multiple-Choice Questions:

6. Which of the following is a key component of effective ethics education programs?
a) Ignoring interactive discussions
b) Using a single teaching method
c) Incorporating case studies, simulations, and role-playing
d) Focusing solely on theoretical knowledge

7. What is an important aspect of professional growth for ethics consultants?
a) Avoiding networking opportunities
b) Pursuing continuing education and certification
c) Limiting participation in professional organizations
d) Ignoring self-care practices

Clinical Vignettes:

8. **Scenario:** Dr. Lee is designing an ethics education program for new healthcare providers. What is the best approach to ensure the program is effective?
a) Use only lectures to convey information
b) Incorporate a variety of teaching methods, including case studies and simulations
c) Focus exclusively on legal aspects of ethics
d) Avoid assessing learning outcomes

9. **Scenario:** Sarah, an ethics consultant, feels overwhelmed by the emotionally challenging nature of her work. What is the best course of action for her to manage stress and avoid burnout?
a) Continue working without any breaks
b) Set boundaries, seek support, and practice self-care
c) Ignore feelings of stress and burnout
d) Increase her workload to keep busy

10. **Scenario:** John, a new ethics consultant, wants to stay current with developments in the field and connect with peers. What is the best approach for him?
a) Avoid attending conferences and workshops
b) Actively engage with professional organizations and seek out continuing education opportunities
c) Limit his involvement in networking activities
d) Rely solely on his initial training for professional development

Correct Answers:

1. True
2. False (Case studies are very useful in illustrating real-world ethical dilemmas. They provide valuable insights into complex situations, helping ethics consultants and healthcare providers learn from real-life scenarios and apply ethical principles effectively.)
3. True
4. False (Networking and participation in professional organizations provide significant benefits for ethics consultants. These activities offer opportunities for professional growth, sharing best practices, staying informed about developments in the field, and connecting with peers.)
5. True
6. c) Incorporating case studies, simulations, and role-playing
7. b) Pursuing continuing education and certification
8. b) Incorporate a variety of teaching methods, including case studies and simulations
9. b) Set boundaries, seek support, and practice self-care
10. b) Actively engage with professional organizations and seek out continuing education opportunities

***

Further Readings and References

- Beauchamp, T. L., & Childress, J. F. (2019). Principles of Biomedical Ethics (8th ed.). Oxford University Press.
  - *This foundational text provides an in-depth discussion of the four principles of biomedical ethics: autonomy, beneficence, nonmaleficence, and justice.*
- Jonsen, A. R., Siegler, M., & Winslade, W. J. (2015). Clinical Ethics: A Practical Approach to Ethical Decisions in Clinical Medicine (8th ed.). McGraw-Hill Education.
  - *A practical guide addressing ethical dilemmas in clinical practice, with case studies and frameworks for decision-making.*
- American Society for Bioethics and Humanities (ASBH). (2011). Core Competencies for Healthcare Ethics Consultation. ASBH.
  - *This document outlines the essential skills and knowledge required for healthcare ethics consultants, emphasizing the role of ethics consultation in clinical practice.*
- Dubler, N. N., & Liebman, C. B. (2011). Bioethics Mediation: A Guide to Shaping Shared Solutions. Vanderbilt University Press.
  - *A guide on using mediation techniques in bioethics consultations to shape shared solutions and resolve conflicts.*
- Fisher, R., Ury, W., & Patton, B. (2011). Getting to Yes: Negotiating Agreement Without Giving In (3rd ed.). Penguin Books.
  - *A classic guide on negotiation and conflict resolution, offering practical strategies for finding mutually acceptable solutions.*
- Halpern, J. (2001). From Detached Concern to Empathy: Humanizing Medical Practice. Oxford University Press.
  - *A book exploring the role of empathy in medical practice, highlighting its importance for building trust and rapport with patients.*

- Campbell, M. L., & Guzman, J. A. (2003). "*Impact of a Proactive Approach to Improve End-of-Life Care in a Medical ICU.*" *Chest*, 123(1), 266-271.
    - *This article explores the impact of proactive end-of-life care planning in intensive care settings, relevant to discussions on advance directives and living wills.*
- Fiester, A. (2007). "*Mediation and Moral Aporia in the Clinical Setting.*" *The American Journal of Bioethics*, 7(2), 23-25.
    - *An article exploring the role of mediation in clinical ethics consultation, highlighting the importance of conflict resolution and moral reflection.*
- Grady, C. (2010). "*Do IRBs Protect Human Research Participants?*" *JAMA*, 304(10), 1122-1123.
    - *This article discusses the role of Institutional Review Boards (IRBs) in protecting human research participants, relevant to the ethics consultation process in research settings.*
- Schyve, P. M. (2007). "*Language Differences as a Barrier to Quality and Safety in Health Care: The Joint Commission Perspective.*" *Journal of General Internal Medicine*, 22(Suppl 2), 360-361.
    - *An article discussing the impact of language and cultural differences on healthcare quality and safety, relevant to the practice of culturally sensitive consultations.*
- Emanuel, E. J., Wendler, D., & Grady, C. (2000). "*What Makes Clinical Research Ethical?*" *JAMA*, 283(20), 2701-2711.
    - *This article outlines the ethical principles guiding clinical research, including informed consent, risk-benefit analysis, and the fair selection of research subjects.*
- Cruess, S. R., & Cruess, R. L. (2006). "*Teaching Professionalism: General Principles.*" *Medical Teacher*, 28(3), 205-208.
    - *An article discussing the general principles of teaching professionalism in medical education, relevant to ethics education and training.*

- Epstein, R. M., & Hundert, E. M. (2002). "*Defining and Assessing Professional Competence.*" *JAMA*, 287(2), 226-235.
  - *This article explores the definition and assessment of professional competence in healthcare, relevant to the development of effective ethics education programs.*
- Fins, J. J., & Bacchetta, M. D. (1995). "*Framing the Clinical Ethics Case Consultation: A Pedagogical and Problem-Oriented Approach.*" *Journal of Clinical Ethics*, 6(3), 239-251.
  - *This article offers a pedagogical approach to conducting ethics consultations, focusing on case framing and problem-solving strategies.*
- Kaldjian, L. C., et al. (2010). "*An Approach to the Evaluation of Ethics Consultation: The Role of Ethics Quality Improvement.*" *The American Journal of Bioethics*, 10(6), 35-37.
  - *An article discussing the evaluation of ethics consultation services and the importance of ethics quality improvement.*
- Post, S. G., Blustein, J., Gordon, E. J., & Mishkin, D. (Eds.). (2007). Handbook for Health Care Ethics Committees. Johns Hopkins University Press.
  - *A practical guide for ethics committees, with chapters on conducting ethics consultations, policy development, and ethics education.*
- Wear, S., & Bickel, J. (2000). Educating for Professionalism: Creating a Culture of Humanism in Medical Education. University of Iowa Press.
  - *A book discussing the importance of creating a culture of humanism and professionalism in medical education, relevant to ethics education and training.*
- Zoloth, L. (2002). Health Care and the Ethics of Encounter: A Jewish Discussion of Social Justice. University of North Carolina Press.
  - *A discussion of social justice in healthcare from a Jewish ethical perspective, relevant to the principle of justice in bioethics.*

- Shapiro, J., Rucker, L., & Robitshek, D. (2006). "*Teaching the Art of Doctoring: An Innovative Medical Student Elective.*" *Medical Education*, 40(4), 293-301.
  - *This article explores an innovative elective course designed to teach medical students the art of doctoring, including empathy, communication, and ethical decision-making.*

***

Appendix

Forms, Templates, Checklists, and Assessments

In this appendix, you will find a comprehensive list of the forms, templates, checklists, and assessments referenced throughout the text. Each item is accompanied by a brief description of its purpose and intended use within the ethics consultation process and related activities.

Purpose and Use: The tools listed below are designed to support ethics consultants, healthcare providers, and administrators in performing their roles effectively and ethically. By providing structured approaches to documentation, communication, facilitation, and professional development, these resources help ensure consistency, thoroughness, and adherence to ethical standards in various aspects of healthcare practice.

How to Use This Appendix:

- **Reference Guide:** Use this appendix as a quick reference to locate the specific tools you need for different stages of the ethics consultation process, from initial intake to follow-up and debriefing.
- **Implementation:** When implementing or adapting these tools in your practice, refer to the corresponding sections in the text for detailed instructions and best practices.
- **Customization:** Each tool can be customized to fit the specific needs of your organization or practice. Consider how the purposes outlined here align with your goals and make adjustments as necessary to enhance their effectiveness.
- **Training and Education:** Incorporate these tools into training programs for ethics consultants and healthcare providers to

ensure consistent application of ethical principles and practices.

By utilizing the forms, templates, checklists, and assessments detailed in this appendix, you can enhance the quality and consistency of your ethics consultations and related activities, ultimately contributing to better patient care and decision-making.

I. Ethics Consultation Tools

2.1 Ethics Consultation Request Form
Purpose: To formally request an ethics consultation, capturing essential information to facilitate a prompt and effective response.

1.1 Ethics Consultation Intake Form
Purpose: To gather all necessary information at the start of an ethics consultation, ensuring that the consultant has a complete understanding of the situation.

2.2 Ethics Consultation Preparation Checklist
Purpose: To guide ethics consultants in preparing for a consultation by ensuring all relevant information is gathered and considered.

1.2 Ethics Consultation Documentation Template (SOAP Format)
Purpose: To ensure thorough and consistent documentation of ethics consultations using the SOAP (Subjective, Objective, Assessment, Plan) format.

2.3 SOAP Notes
Purpose: To provide a comprehensive and structured format for documenting ethics consultations using the SOAP (Subjective, Objective, Assessment, Plan) method.

2.4 SOAP Notes—Cue Card
Purpose: Quick reference guide for SOAP Notes during consultations.

2.5 Ethics Consultation Follow-Up Checklist
Purpose: To ensure that the recommendations from an ethics consultation are implemented and to monitor their outcomes.

2.6 Ethics Consultation Report Template
Purpose: To create a clear, comprehensive, and concise report summarizing the ethics consultation and its outcomes.

1.3 Ethics Consultation Debrief Checklist
Purpose: To guide a structured debriefing session after an ethics consultation, helping the team reflect on the process, decisions made, and areas for improvement.

II. Communication, Facilitation, and Cultural Competence

3.1 Active Listening and Empathy Checklist
Purpose: To guide ethics consultants in practicing active listening and empathy during consultations, ensuring that all stakeholders feel heard and understood.

3.2 Facilitating Difficult Conversations Template
Purpose: To provide a structured approach to managing difficult conversations in ethics consultations, ensuring a respectful and constructive dialogue.

3.3 Conflict Resolution and Mediation Checklist
Purpose: To guide ethics consultants through the process of mediating conflicts and resolving disputes among patients, families, and healthcare providers.

3.4 Systematic Ethical Analysis Worksheet
Purpose: To help ethics consultants systematically analyze ethical dilemmas using a structured approach, ensuring comprehensive consideration of all relevant factors.

3.5 Cultural Competence Consultation Guide
Purpose: To ensure that ethics consultants approach each

consultation with cultural competence and sensitivity, respecting diverse values and beliefs.

3.6 Interprofessional Collaboration Checklist
Purpose: To guide ethics consultants in effectively collaborating with interprofessional healthcare teams, ensuring integrated and comprehensive ethical decision-making.

III. Specialized Ethics Consultations

4.1 Advance Directives and Living Wills Checklist
Purpose: To guide ethics consultants in discussing and respecting advance directives and living wills, ensuring that patient wishes are honored.

4.2 Palliative Care and Hospice Ethics Consultation Template
Purpose: To ensure that ethical issues in palliative care and hospice are addressed comprehensively, respecting patient autonomy and quality of life.

4.3 Informed Consent and Capacity Assessment Form
Purpose: To assist ethics consultants in evaluating and documenting informed consent and decisional capacity, ensuring patient autonomy is respected.

4.4 Confidentiality and Privacy Checklist
Purpose: To ensure that patient confidentiality is protected and that sensitive information is managed ethically and legally.

4.5 Resource Allocation and Justice Ethics Consultation Template
Purpose: To guide ethics consultants in addressing ethical issues related to resource allocation and ensuring fair and equitable decisions.

4.6 Research Ethics Consultation Checklist
Purpose: To guide ethics consultants in evaluating and addressing ethical issues in clinical research, ensuring participant protection and ethical integrity.

IV. Education and Professional Development

5.1 Ethics Education Program Design Template

Purpose: To guide ethics consultants in designing comprehensive and effective ethics education programs for healthcare providers.

5.2 Professional Development Plan for Ethics Consultants

Purpose: To support the ongoing professional growth of ethics consultants through structured planning and goal-setting.

5.3 Case Study Analysis and Reflection Worksheet

Purpose: To guide ethics consultants and learners in analyzing and reflecting on ethical dilemmas presented in case studies.

5.4 Self-Care Checklist for Ethics Consultants

Purpose: To ensure that ethics consultants maintain their well-being and resilience while working in emotionally challenging environments.

***

Glossary

A

Abortion

Abortion has long been a contentious issue, balancing a woman's autonomy against the rights of the fetus. In the United States, the 1973 Roe v. Wade decision established a woman's right to abortion before viability, based on privacy rights, while the 2022 Dobbs ruling left regulation to individual states. Ethical dilemmas include patient autonomy, ensuring informed consent, minimizing harm, and ensuring equitable access to abortion services. Healthcare providers must navigate moral challenges, conscientious objections, and legal complexities while prioritizing ethical standards such as autonomy, beneficence, nonmaleficence, and justice.

Abuse

Abuse, in its various forms—physical, emotional, sexual, and neglect—presents significant ethical and legal challenges in healthcare. Key dilemmas include balancing patient confidentiality with mandatory reporting laws, respecting patient autonomy while ensuring their safety, and navigating cultural sensitivities. Healthcare providers must prioritize autonomy, beneficence, nonmaleficence, and justice, ensuring victims receive compassionate care and protection from further harm. Mandatory reporting, legal requirements, and ethical obligations intersect in complex ways, requiring healthcare professionals to carefully balance their duties while advocating for the equitable treatment of all victims and supporting their recovery and well-being.

Active Listening

Active listening is a communication technique that involves fully concentrating, understanding, responding, and remembering what the speaker is saying. It requires the listener to engage with the speaker both verbally and non-verbally, demonstrating interest through eye contact, nodding, and appropriate body language. Active listening goes beyond merely hearing words; it involves reflecting back on what is being said, asking clarifying questions, and providing feedback that shows understanding. This approach fosters trust, ensures accurate comprehension, and helps build strong relationships, making it an essential skill in healthcare, counseling, and everyday interpersonal interactions. Active listening promotes empathy, reduces misunderstandings, and supports effective problem-solving, directly aligning with patient-centered care and respecting patient autonomy.

- *Cross-reference: Patient Autonomy, Cultural Competence, Practitioner-Patient Relationship*

Addressing Oneself and Patient

The way healthcare providers introduce themselves and address patients is crucial for building trust and respect. Traditionally, formal introductions using titles like "Dr." maintain professional boundaries, while patient-centered care emphasizes familiarity. Key dilemmas include balancing formality and informality, respecting cultural expectations, managing power dynamics, and honoring patient preferences. Providers must be sensitive to how they address patients, respecting their autonomy while fostering trust and ensuring fairness. Legal and institutional policies influence these interactions, and ethical principles like beneficence, nonmaleficence, and justice guide the appropriate way to address patients in healthcare settings.

Advance Directives

Advance directives provide individuals with a legal means to express their medical treatment preferences when they can no longer communicate. These documents, including living wills and durable powers of attorney for healthcare, raise ethical challenges such as balancing patient autonomy with clinical judgment, addressing outdated directives, and resolving interpretation disputes. Surrogate decision-making and cultural considerations further complicate these situations. Healthcare providers must respect advance directives while adhering to legal requirements, institutional policies, and ethical principles like beneficence, nonmaleficence, and justice, ensuring that patient wishes align with medical standards and promote patient well-being.

- *Cross-reference: Living Will, Durable Power of Attorney (DPOA), Surrogate Decision-Making, Patient Autonomy, Informed Consent*

Alternative Therapy

A treatment or therapeutic approach that falls outside conventional medical practices, such as acupuncture or herbal medicine. When a patient expresses interest in an alternative therapy that diverges from medical standards of care, the practitioner should first seek to understand the patient's reasons for this interest. This allows for open communication and helps the practitioner provide informed and patient-centered care while ensuring that such therapies do not interfere with standard treatments.

Artificial Intelligence in Healthcare

Artificial Intelligence (AI) in healthcare refers to the use of advanced algorithms and machine learning techniques to analyze complex medical data, improve diagnostics, personalize treatment plans, and enhance patient care. AI's ability to process vast amounts of information quickly can lead to early detection of diseases, optimized treatment options, and efficient resource allocation. However, its integration raises ethical concerns about patient autonomy, privacy, and data security. Issues of algorithmic bias, accountability for AI-driven decisions, and the potential erosion of the patient-practitioner relationship must be addressed to ensure that AI applications align with the principles of beneficence, nonmaleficence, autonomy, and justice.

- *Cross-reference: Data Analytics, Patient Autonomy, Confidentiality, Ethical Decision-Making*

Assisted Death

Assisted death, including physician-assisted suicide (PAS) and euthanasia, raises ethical, legal, and professional dilemmas. Balancing patient autonomy with healthcare providers' ethical commitments to healing is a central issue. Ethical concerns include the potential for coercion in vulnerable populations, cultural and religious differences, and the slippery slope argument. Legal frameworks vary by state, with some allowing PAS under strict conditions. Providers must navigate these complexities while adhering to legal requirements, institutional policies, and the principles of beneficence, nonmaleficence, and justice. Providers must prioritize comprehensive palliative care and uphold ethical standards while respecting patients' end-of-life decisions.

Autonomy

Autonomy is the ethical principle that recognizes the right of patients to make informed, voluntary decisions about their healthcare. For autonomy to be respected, the practitioner must ensure that informed consent has been obtained, meaning that the patient or surrogate possesses the decisional capacity to understand their diagnosis, prognosis, and all available treatment options, including their associated benefits and risks. Respecting autonomy includes honoring a patient's choice even when it contradicts medical advice, provided the decision is reasonable and complies with legal and ethical standards. The decision must be made free from coercion, reflecting the patient's reasonable goals, values, and priorities while adhering to medical standards, institutional policies, and legal requirements. The final decision should be communicated clearly, documented in the medical records, and shared with all relevant healthcare team members.

- *Cross-reference: Informed Consent, Capacity, Substituted Judgment, Advance Directive*

B

Balance (Weigh and Balance)

The Weigh and Balance process in ethical decision-making involves both the patient or surrogate and the practitioner collaboratively assessing the relative importance of the four primary bioethical principles: autonomy, beneficence, nonmaleficence, and justice. In the Weigh phase, they determine the weight of each principle based on the patient's reasonable goals, values, and priorities, while also considering medical standards of care, institutional policies, and legal mandates. In the Balance phase, they decide which principle or combination of principles should guide the decision-making process, aiming to arrive at a rational and reasonable recommendation that aligns with the patient's best interests and ethical obligations.

- *Cross-reference: Autonomy, Beneficence, Nonmaleficence, Justice, Ethics Consultation*

Belmont Report

The Belmont Report, published in 1979 by the National Commission for the Protection of Human Subjects of Biomedical and Behavioral Research, is a foundational document in the field of bioethics. It outlines ethical principles and guidelines for research involving human subjects, emphasizing respect for persons, beneficence, and justice. The report advocates for obtaining informed consent from participants, assessing risks and benefits to minimize harm, and ensuring equitable selection of subjects. These principles have shaped regulations and practices for ethical conduct in research, providing a framework to protect the rights and welfare of human subjects in biomedical and behavioral studies.

Beneficence

Beneficence is the ethical obligation for healthcare providers to act in the best interest of the patient, prioritizing their well-being and quality of life. To fulfill this duty, practitioners must present treatment options that align with the patient's reasonable goals, values, and priorities, ensuring that these options maximize the patient's benefits. All proposed treatments must comply with established medical standards of care, institutional policies, and legal mandates. Furthermore, the practitioner should regularly review and adjust treatment decisions to reflect any changes in the patient's condition or circumstances, ensuring that beneficence continues to guide patient care.

- *Cross-reference: Nonmaleficence, Justice, Autonomy, Weigh and Balance*

Best Interests

The concept of patient best interest refers to the guiding principle in healthcare decision-making that prioritizes the health, well-being, and overall welfare of the patient. Decisions are made based on what is most beneficial for the patient, considering their medical needs, personal values, and reasonable goals. This principle involves evaluating the potential benefits and burdens of treatment options, including the likelihood of achieving desired health outcomes, quality of life, and minimizing suffering. It requires healthcare providers to act with compassion, respect patient autonomy, and adhere to medical standards of care, institutional policies, and legal requirements.

Best Practices

Best practices are the established methods, procedures, and guidelines that are widely accepted as being the most effective and efficient ways to achieve desired outcomes in a specific field or industry. These practices are typically based on research, evidence, and expert consensus, and they serve as benchmarks for quality and performance. In healthcare, best practices aim to improve patient care, enhance safety, and optimize resource use by adhering to proven standards of clinical excellence. Organizations and professionals adopt best practices to ensure consistency, minimize risks, and maintain high standards of service, thereby promoting optimal outcomes and continuous improvement..

Bioethics Committee

A bioethics committee is a interprofession group that provides guidance and recommendations on ethical issues related to healthcare, medical research, and clinical practices. Comprised of healthcare professionals, ethicists, legal experts, and community representatives, these committees play a crucial role in addressing complex ethical dilemmas, such as end-of-life decisions, patient consent, allocation of scarce resources, and confidentiality. Bioethics committees review cases, develop ethical policies, and provide education and support to healthcare staff and patients. By promoting ethical standards and facilitating thoughtful deliberation, bioethics committees help ensure that patient care and medical practices align with ethical principles, legal requirements, and societal values.

Bioethics Program Director

A Bioethics Program Director is a leadership role responsible for overseeing and managing an institution's bioethics program. This position involves developing and implementing policies, guidelines, and educational initiatives that address ethical issues in healthcare, research, and clinical practice. The director provides expertise and guidance on complex ethical dilemmas, facilitates ethics consultations, and ensures that ethical standards align with institutional policies, medical standards of care, and legal requirements. Additionally, the Bioethics Program Director often collaborates with healthcare professionals, administrators, and ethics committees to promote ethical decision-making, enhance patient care, and uphold the institution's commitment to ethical integrity and compliance..

Bioethics

Bioethics is a multidisciplinary field that examines the ethical, legal, and social implications of advancements in biology, medicine, and healthcare. It addresses complex issues such as patient autonomy, informed consent, end-of-life care, reproductive rights, genetic engineering, and the allocation of scarce medical resources. Bioethics seeks to guide decision-making by applying ethical principles, such as autonomy, beneficence, nonmaleficence, and justice, to real-world dilemmas faced by patients, healthcare professionals, researchers, and policymakers. The field promotes the development of ethical guidelines, policies, and practices to ensure that biomedical and healthcare innovations are conducted in a morally responsible and socially just manner.

C

Capacity

Capacity refers to an individual's ability to understand, appreciate, and make informed decisions about their own healthcare. It involves assessing whether a person can comprehend the nature and consequences of a particular medical decision, including the benefits, risks, and alternatives. Capacity is a crucial component of informed consent and can vary depending on the complexity of the decision and the individual's cognitive and emotional state. It is not a fixed trait but can fluctuate over time and in different situations. Healthcare professionals are responsible for evaluating capacity, ensuring that patients can make autonomous and reasoned decisions about their treatment options.

- *Cross-reference: Informed Consent, Patient Autonomy, Surrogate Decision-Making, Mental Health*

Capital Punishment

Capital punishment, or the death penalty, remains a contentious issue, raising ethical, legal, and social concerns. Ethical dilemmas include balancing justice with retribution, the risk of wrongful convictions, and whether execution methods violate the Eighth Amendment's prohibition against cruel and unusual punishment. Racial and socioeconomic disparities further complicate its fair application. Healthcare professionals face ethical conflicts when asked to participate in executions, as their role prioritizes healing, not harm. The principles of beneficence, nonmaleficence, and justice call for opposition to capital punishment and advocacy for humane treatment and fairness in the justice system.

Case Consultation

Case consultation is a process in healthcare ethics where a team of interdisciplinary professionals evaluates and provides guidance on complex ethical dilemmas arising in patient care. These consultations typically involve reviewing the patient's medical information, understanding the ethical issues at stake, and considering the perspectives of all involved parties, including patients, families, and healthcare providers. The goal is to reach a consensus that respects patient autonomy, adheres to ethical principles like beneficence, nonmaleficence, and justice, and complies with legal and institutional standards. Case consultations aim to support ethical decision-making, enhance patient care, and resolve conflicts in a fair and transparent manner.

Case Studies

Case studies are in-depth analyses of real-world or hypothetical scenarios used to explore complex issues in a specific context, often within education, healthcare, law, or business. In bioethics, case studies serve as valuable tools for examining ethical dilemmas, illustrating how ethical principles can be applied to real-life situations involving patient care and medical decision-making. By providing a detailed account of a particular situation, including background information, challenges, and possible resolutions, case studies help learners and practitioners develop critical thinking skills, understand the nuances of ethical principles, and prepare for similar situations in their professional practice.

Chaperones

The use of chaperones in clinical settings involves balancing patient privacy with the need for protection during sensitive examinations. While chaperones help prevent misconduct and provide reassurance, they may infringe on a patient's comfort and autonomy. Patients have the right to accept or refuse a chaperone, and healthcare providers must clearly explain their role. Cultural considerations, legal liability, and institutional policies also influence chaperone use. Ethical principles like beneficence, nonmaleficence, and justice guide the fair and respectful implementation of chaperones, ensuring patient comfort and safety while adhering to legal and institutional mandates.

Checklists

Checklists are structured tools used in various settings, including healthcare, to ensure that tasks are completed systematically and consistently. In clinical environments, checklists help healthcare providers follow standard protocols, enhance patient safety, and minimize errors by providing a clear, step-by-step outline of necessary actions. They serve as reminders for critical tasks, such as verifying patient identity, confirming medication dosages, or following specific procedural steps. Checklists are also used in ethical decision-making to ensure that all relevant ethical principles, legal mandates, and patient preferences are considered. Their use promotes thoroughness, accountability, and quality assurance in healthcare practices.

Clinical Ethics Committees

A Clinical Ethics Committee is a multidisciplinary group within a healthcare institution that provides guidance on ethical issues arising in patient care. These committees typically consist of healthcare professionals, ethicists, legal advisors, and sometimes patient representatives, working collaboratively to analyze complex ethical dilemmas, offer recommendations, and support healthcare providers and patients in making informed, ethical decisions. Clinical Ethics Committees help ensure that patient care aligns with ethical standards, institutional policies, and legal requirements by facilitating case consultations, developing ethical guidelines, and providing education and training on bioethics to healthcare staff. Their role is critical in promoting ethical integrity and patient-centered care in healthcare settings.

Clinical Ethics Consultation

A Clinical Ethics Consultation is a service provided by ethics experts within healthcare settings to address and resolve ethical dilemmas that arise in patient care. These consultations involve analyzing specific cases to clarify ethical issues, providing recommendations, and facilitating communication among patients, families, and healthcare teams. The goal of a clinical ethics consultation is to support informed, ethical decision-making that aligns with the patient's values, medical standards of care, and legal and institutional policies. By offering guidance on complex ethical situations, clinical ethics consultations help ensure that patient care is both ethically sound and compassionate.

Clinical Vignettes

Clinical vignettes are brief, descriptive scenarios that present a medical or ethical dilemma encountered in clinical practice. They are used as educational tools to facilitate learning and discussion among healthcare professionals, students, and ethics committees. By depicting realistic patient cases, clinical vignettes help illustrate complex medical conditions, ethical challenges, and decision-making processes, allowing participants to apply theoretical knowledge to practical situations. These narratives often include details about the patient's medical history, symptoms, and the ethical issues involved, encouraging critical thinking, problem-solving, and the application of ethical principles and best practices in a controlled, reflective environment..

Confidentiality

Confidentiality is a cornerstone of the patient-provider relationship, ensuring the privacy of personal health information (PHI). Ethical dilemmas arise when maintaining confidentiality conflicts with public safety, legal requirements, or the patient's welfare. Balancing patient privacy with obligations to disclose in situations like reporting infectious diseases or abuse is complex. Legal frameworks like HIPAA govern confidentiality practices, and unauthorized disclosures can harm patient trust. Healthcare providers must protect patient information while ensuring their actions align with ethical principles like autonomy, beneficence, nonmaleficence, and justice, respecting patients' reasonable goals and complying with legal standards.

Conflict of Interest

A conflict of interest arises when a healthcare professional's personal, financial, or other secondary interests could compromise their professional judgment and commitment to the patient's best interests. Conflicts may occur in relationships with the pharmaceutical industry, clinical research, or dual administrative roles. Ethical dilemmas center on transparency, maintaining impartiality, and balancing personal interests with professional responsibilities. Healthcare providers must disclose potential conflicts to maintain patient trust, uphold autonomy, and ensure that care aligns with ethical principles like beneficence, nonmaleficence, and justice. Managing conflicts ethically preserves the integrity of patient care and complies with legal standards.

Consent, Minors

Consent for minors refers to the legal and ethical requirement to obtain permission from a parent or legal guardian for medical treatment or participation in research involving individuals under a certain age, typically 18 years. Because minors are generally considered not to have the full legal capacity to make informed healthcare decisions, parents or guardians must provide consent on their behalf. In some cases, minors can consent to their own treatment, especially if they are deemed "mature minors," or in situations involving reproductive health, mental health services, or treatment for substance abuse, depending on state laws and regulations.

Continuing Education

Continuing education refers to the ongoing professional development activities that individuals engage in to maintain, enhance, and expand their knowledge, skills, and competencies throughout their careers. In the healthcare field, continuing education is essential for keeping up-to-date with the latest medical research, technological advancements, and evolving best practices. It often involves attending workshops, conferences, courses, and seminars, as well as completing online training and certifications. By participating in continuing education, healthcare professionals can ensure they provide high-quality, evidence-based care, meet licensure requirements, and adapt to changes in their respective fields, ultimately improving patient outcomes and advancing their professional expertise.

Contraception

Contraception has been central to debates around reproductive rights, autonomy, and healthcare access. Ethical dilemmas arise from religious and moral opposition, disparities in access, and ensuring informed consent. Healthcare providers must balance respecting patient autonomy, providing comprehensive contraceptive options, and minimizing harm while adhering to ethical principles like beneficence, nonmaleficence, and justice. Ensuring equitable access to contraception, particularly for vulnerable populations, and navigating legal and cultural considerations are critical. Managing these complexities requires aligning care with the patient's reasonable goals, values, and priorities within the framework of medical standards and legal mandates

CRISPR Gene Editing

CRISPR gene editing is a revolutionary technology that enables precise alterations to DNA, offering the potential to correct genetic disorders, prevent diseases, and enhance human traits. While it holds promise for treating conditions like cystic fibrosis and sickle cell anemia, its use raises significant ethical concerns. Issues include the potential for unintended genetic changes, the long-term impacts on future generations, and the ethical implications of editing human embryos. CRISPR also poses questions about consent, accessibility, and equity in healthcare. To navigate these challenges, its application must align with ethical principles of autonomy, beneficence, nonmaleficence, and justice.

- *Cross-reference: Genetic Information Nondiscrimination Act (GINA), Patient Autonomy, Informed Consent, Ethical Decision-Making*

Cultural Competence

Cultural competence is the ability of healthcare providers and organizations to understand, respect, and effectively interact with patients from diverse cultural backgrounds. This competence involves recognizing the cultural beliefs, values, and practices that influence a patient's health behaviors and decisions. Culturally competent care requires healthcare professionals to be aware of their own cultural biases, acquire knowledge about different cultural perspectives, and develop skills to communicate and deliver care that respects patients' cultural preferences. The goal of cultural competence is to improve patient outcomes, enhance patient satisfaction, and reduce health disparities by ensuring that care is responsive to the cultural and linguistic needs of all patients.

D

Data Analytics

Data analytics involves the systematic computational analysis of data to uncover patterns, correlations, and insights that can inform decision-making processes. In healthcare, data analytics is used to analyze patient data, clinical outcomes, operational efficiency, and other key performance indicators. By employing techniques such as statistical analysis, machine learning, and predictive modeling, healthcare professionals can identify trends, optimize treatment plans, enhance patient care, and reduce costs. Data analytics also plays a crucial role in public health for tracking disease outbreaks, improving population health management, and supporting evidence-based policy decisions. The ultimate goal is to leverage data to improve health outcomes and operational effectiveness.

Death with Dignity — Assisted Dying

"Death with Dignity" refers to laws allowing terminally ill patients to request life-ending medication to die on their own terms. Ethical dilemmas arise from balancing patient autonomy with moral, religious, and legal opposition, while protecting vulnerable populations from coercion. Healthcare providers must navigate complex issues such as beneficence, nonmaleficence, and justice, ensuring informed, voluntary decisions. Legal permissibility varies across states, but it does not determine professional standards. Upholding patient rights while adhering to ethical guidelines is crucial for maintaining the integrity of healthcare and public trust.

Decision-Making Capacity
Decision-making capacity refers to an individual's ability to understand, evaluate, and make informed decisions about their own medical care. This involves the ability to comprehend relevant information about a condition and its treatment options, appreciate the consequences of various choices, reason through the options in a logical and coherent manner, and communicate a clear and consistent choice. Assessing decision-making capacity is crucial in healthcare, especially when patients face complex medical decisions or when consent for treatment is required. A patient's capacity may be influenced by factors such as mental health conditions, cognitive impairments, or the effects of medications, and it can vary over time.

Declaration of Geneva
The Declaration of Geneva, adopted by the World Medical Association (WMA) in 1948, is a modern restatement of the Hippocratic Oath, outlining the ethical duties of physicians. It was created in response to the atrocities committed during World War II, emphasizing the physician's role in preserving human life and dignity. The Declaration pledges respect for human life, dedication to serving humanity, and a commitment to the principles of medical ethics, regardless of a patient's status, race, religion, or nationality. It has been revised over time to address contemporary issues in medical ethics, such as patient autonomy, confidentiality,

and the importance of treating patients with respect and compassion.

Deontological Ethics

Deontological ethics is a moral theory that emphasizes the importance of following ethical principles and duties regardless of the consequences. Rooted in the works of Immanuel Kant, this approach argues that actions are morally right or wrong based on their adherence to rules, duties, or obligations rather than their outcomes. According to deontological ethics, certain actions are intrinsically right or wrong, and individuals have a moral duty to act according to these principles. This theory prioritizes the adherence to moral laws or duties, such as honesty or justice, over the pursuit of overall good or utility.

Digital Health Ethics

Digital health ethics encompasses the ethical considerations surrounding the use of digital technologies in healthcare, such as mobile health apps, telemedicine, wearable devices, and electronic health records. Key ethical issues include safeguarding patient privacy, ensuring data security, maintaining the integrity and accuracy of digital health information, and managing consent for data collection and use. There are also concerns about equitable access to digital health tools, potential biases in algorithms, and the impact on the patient-practitioner relationship. To address these challenges, digital health practices must adhere to ethical principles of autonomy, beneficence, nonmaleficence, and justice.

- *Cross-reference: Electronic Health Records (EHR), Patient Autonomy, Confidentiality, Telemedicine*

Disagreement — Attending vs Resident

Disagreements between attending physicians and residents are common in healthcare, reflecting the dynamic between experienced professionals and those in training. While attendings hold ultimate responsibility for patient care, residents contribute fresh perspectives informed by recent training. Ethical dilemmas arise when opinions diverge on diagnoses, treatment options, or patient autonomy, often complicated by the need to align with medical standards, institutional policies, and legal mandates. Balancing respect for resident input with patient-centered care requires clear communication, mutual respect, and adherence to bioethical principles like autonomy, beneficence, nonmaleficence, and justice. Managing disagreements effectively ensures patient safety and professional growth.

Do-Not-Resuscitate Orders (DNR)
Do-Not-Resuscitate (DNR) orders allow patients to refuse cardiopulmonary resuscitation (CPR) in situations where resuscitation may not align with their values or prognosis. These orders balance the ethical principles of autonomy, beneficence, nonmaleficence, and justice, allowing patients to make informed decisions about their end-of-life care. Ethical dilemmas often arise from the tension between respecting patient autonomy and healthcare providers' duty to preserve life. Proper documentation, clear communication, and consideration of legal and ethical guidelines are crucial to ensuring that DNR orders are respected, thus promoting patient dignity and avoiding unnecessary harm.

Doctrine of Double Effect
The Doctrine of Double Effect (DDE) is a moral principle asserting that an action with both good and bad effects is permissible if the intent behind the action is to achieve the good effect, with the bad effect being a foreseen but unintended consequence. Originating from Thomas Aquinas' Natural Law tradition, DDE is often invoked in healthcare to justify treatments that alleviate suffering but may hasten death. Modern bioethics challenges DDE for its focus on practitioner intention, arguing that it inadequately addresses the need for patient autonomy and informed consent, which are foundational to ethical medical practice today.

Durable Power of Attorney (DPOA)
A Durable Power of Attorney is a legal document that grants a

designated individual, known as the agent or attorney-in-fact, the authority to make decisions on behalf of the principal (the person granting the power) if they become incapacitated or unable to make decisions for themselves. Unlike a regular Power of Attorney, a DPOA remains effective even if the principal loses mental capacity. This document can cover a broad range of matters, including financial, legal, and healthcare decisions. In healthcare contexts, a DPOA for healthcare allows the agent to make medical decisions according to the principal's wishes, values, and best interests

---

E

Electronic Health Records (EHR)
Electronic Health Records (EHR) are digital versions of patients' paper charts, encompassing comprehensive and real-time data about a patient's medical history, diagnoses, medications, treatment plans, immunization dates, allergies, radiology images, and laboratory test results. EHRs are designed to be accessed by authorized healthcare providers and staff across different healthcare settings, facilitating coordinated care and improving the quality and safety of patient care. They also support clinical decision-making by integrating evidence-based tools and guidelines. EHRs enhance communication, streamline workflows, and contribute to more accurate and efficient healthcare delivery, while also safeguarding patient privacy through secure access protocols..

Email and Electronic Communication
Email and electronic communication have transformed healthcare by offering speed and efficiency in patient-provider interactions. However, these methods present ethical and legal concerns, particularly regarding patient privacy, data security, and informed consent. The Health Insurance Portability and Accountability Act

(HIPAA) mandates that communications containing Protected Health Information (PHI) be HIPAA-compliant, leading many providers to use secure patient portals rather than traditional email. These portals enhance patient privacy, ensure legal compliance, and maintain accountability. While electronic communication improves accessibility, healthcare providers must balance the benefits with the need to protect patient information and uphold ethical standards like autonomy and nonmaleficence.

Emergency Medical Treatment and Labor Act (EMTALA)
The Emergency Medical Treatment and Labor Act (EMTALA) is a federal law enacted in 1986 that requires hospitals with emergency departments to provide emergency medical care to anyone needing treatment, regardless of their insurance status, ability to pay, or citizenship. Under EMTALA, hospitals must conduct a medical screening to determine if an emergency medical condition exists and provide stabilizing treatment if necessary. If a hospital is unable to stabilize a patient, it must arrange for a proper transfer to another facility that can provide the necessary care. EMTALA is a critical safeguard to ensure access to emergency medical services and prevent patient dumping.

Errors
Errors in healthcare pose ethical and legal concerns, impacting patient safety, provider integrity, and trust in the healthcare system. Key dilemmas include transparency, disclosure, and accountability. Historically, providers feared litigation or damage to reputation from disclosing errors, but modern ethical standards demand openness to respect patient autonomy. Failure to disclose errors violates patients' rights, undermines informed consent, and may result in legal consequences. Ethical principles such as beneficence, nonmaleficence, and justice require that errors be disclosed to prevent harm, improve patient safety, and ensure fair treatment for all. Transparency fosters trust and supports ethical, patient-centered care.

Ethics Consultant

An ethics consultant is a professional who provides expertise in ethical decision-making within healthcare settings. Their role involves offering guidance on complex ethical issues, helping to resolve conflicts, and ensuring that patient care aligns with ethical principles such as autonomy, beneficence, nonmaleficence, and justice. Ethics consultants work closely with patients, families, and healthcare teams to facilitate communication, clarify ethical dilemmas, and recommend ethically appropriate actions. They may also contribute to policy development, education, and training within their institutions. Ethics consultants are vital in promoting ethical standards and enhancing the quality of care in healthcare organizations..

Ethics Consultation

Ethics consultation is a process through which healthcare professionals, patients, or their families seek guidance on complex ethical issues that arise in clinical practice. The purpose of ethics consultation is to support informed and ethical decision-making, ensuring that patient care aligns with ethical principles such as autonomy, beneficence, nonmaleficence, and justice. During an ethics consultation, an ethics consultant or ethics committee reviews the case, engages with the relevant stakeholders, and provides recommendations to help resolve ethical dilemmas. These consultations play a crucial role in addressing conflicts, clarifying values, and promoting ethically sound practices in healthcare settings.

Ethics Rounds

Ethics rounds are structured discussions held within healthcare settings where a multidisciplinary team of healthcare professionals, including physicians, nurses, social workers, and ethics consultants, gather to review and analyze ethical issues related to patient care. These rounds provide a forum for team members to discuss challenging cases, reflect on ethical dilemmas, and explore the application of ethical principles such as autonomy, beneficence, nonmaleficence, and justice. Ethics rounds contribute to the ongoing education of healthcare providers, promote an ethical culture within healthcare organizations, and support ethical decision-making by integrating ethical considerations into clinical practice.

- *Cross-reference: Ethics Consultation, Clinical Ethics Committees, Case Consultation*

Euthanasia

Euthanasia, the intentional ending of a person's life by a healthcare professional to alleviate suffering, raises significant ethical, legal, and philosophical challenges. The practice is illegal in the United States, where end-of-life care focuses on alternatives like palliative care. Key ethical dilemmas include balancing patient autonomy, the sanctity of life, and the physician's duty to do no harm. While some argue for euthanasia as an act of compassion, professional guidelines reject it, emphasizing patient care through legally and ethically accepted means like pain management and hospice. The debate centers on respecting life, patient rights, and ethical boundaries.

F

Financial Disclosures

Financial disclosures in healthcare involve the transparent reporting of financial relationships between healthcare providers and external entities, such as pharmaceutical companies or medical device manufacturers. These disclosures are essential to avoiding conflicts of interest, ensuring patient trust, and maintaining the integrity of clinical decision-making. The Physician Payments Sunshine Act mandates transparency in these relationships, aiming to prevent undue influence on patient care. Ethical guidelines from organizations like the AMA emphasize the need for financial transparency to protect patient welfare, uphold autonomy, and ensure that medical decisions are free from bias.

Four Principles — Principlism

This foundational framework of biomedical ethics guides ethical decision-making by emphasizing four key principles. Patient Autonomy (Informed Consent): This principle respects the rights of patients to make informed decisions about their own healthcare based on their goals, values, and priorities. Practitioner Beneficence (Maximize Benefits): It focuses on acting in the patient's best interests to promote their well-being and enhance their quality of life. Practitioner Nonmaleficence (Minimize Burdens): This principle is about avoiding harm and minimizing the burdens of treatment on the patient. Public Justice (Ensure Fairness): It ensures that fairness and equity are upheld in the distribution of healthcare resources and treatment options.

Futile Treatment

Futile treatment refers to medical interventions that are unlikely to benefit the patient, particularly in end-of-life situations. This concept raises ethical dilemmas regarding patient autonomy, healthcare providers' professional judgment, and the allocation of resources. While patients or families may request continued treatment, healthcare professionals must balance these requests with the ethical duty to avoid administering ineffective care. Futile treatment often involves conflicts over the definition of "benefit" and requires clear communication to align care with the patient's reasonable goals, values, and priorities, while upholding ethical principles such as beneficence, nonmaleficence, and justice.

G

Genetic Information Nondiscrimination Act (GINA)

The Genetic Information Nondiscrimination Act (GINA) of 2008 prohibits the misuse of genetic information in health insurance and employment. It protects individuals from discrimination based on genetic predispositions to certain diseases. GINA ensures that genetic data cannot be used by employers or insurers to make decisions about hiring, coverage, or premiums. By safeguarding privacy and promoting fairness, GINA supports patient autonomy and encourages genetic testing without fear of negative repercussions, fostering public trust in personalized medicine. This legislation aligns with the ethical principles of nonmaleficence, beneficence, justice, and respect for patient autonomy.

Gift Acceptance

Gift acceptance in healthcare involves ethical considerations surrounding the influence of gifts on medical judgment and patient care. While gifts were historically seen as expressions of gratitude, contemporary concerns focus on the potential for gifts from patients or commercial entities to affect clinical decisions. Accepting gifts may blur professional boundaries and create conflicts of interest, undermining trust and patient autonomy. Ethical guidelines, such as those from the AMA, advise against accepting gifts that could influence decision-making, prioritizing transparency, fairness, and the patient's best interests to maintain professional integrity and uphold ethical standards in patient care.

Gunshot Wounds and Mandatory Reporting

Gunshot wounds (GSWs) present ethical and legal challenges for healthcare providers, particularly due to mandatory reporting laws that require disclosing GSW incidents to law enforcement. These laws aim to protect public safety but can conflict with patient privacy and autonomy. Healthcare providers must balance their duty to report with ethical obligations to maintain confidentiality, minimize harm, and ensure justice. Reporting only the minimum required information and being transparent with patients about these legal requirements helps to maintain trust while adhering to public safety regulations, aligning with the ethical principles of autonomy, beneficence, nonmaleficence, and justice.

H

Health Insurance Portability and Accountability Act (HIPAA)
The Health Insurance Portability and Accountability Act (HIPAA) is a U.S. federal law enacted in 1996 that aims to protect the privacy and security of individuals' medical information. HIPAA establishes national standards for the handling, storage, and transmission of protected health information (PHI), ensuring that patient data remains confidential and secure. The law also grants patients rights over their health information, including the right to access their medical records and request corrections. Additionally, HIPAA includes provisions that facilitate the portability of health insurance coverage for individuals transitioning between jobs, thereby protecting health coverage continuity

Healthcare Standards of Care
Standard of care refers to the level and quality of care that a reasonably competent healthcare professional, with a similar background and in a similar community, would provide under comparable circumstances. It serves as a benchmark for assessing the appropriateness and effectiveness of medical treatment and interventions. The standard of care is determined by various factors, including clinical guidelines, expert opinions, medical literature, and prevailing practices. Adherence to the standard of care ensures that patients receive safe and effective treatment, while deviations from this standard may lead to medical liability or malpractice claims if harm results

Hippocratic Oath
The Hippocratic Oath is a seminal ethical code of conduct historically attributed to the ancient Greek physician Hippocrates and serves as a foundational text for medical ethics. Traditionally taken by physicians, the Oath commits them to practicing medicine ethically and honestly, emphasizing principles such as patient confidentiality, nonmaleficence "*do no harm*" and beneficence

(acting in the patient's best interests). It includes commitments to avoid causing harm or injustice, refraining from exploiting patients, and upholding professional integrity. While the Oath has evolved over centuries, its core tenets continue to influence contemporary medical ethics and guide healthcare professionals in their practice.

Hospice Care
Hospice care provides comfort and support for patients with terminal illnesses, focusing on improving quality of life rather than curing illness. It involves symptom management, emotional support, and addressing the spiritual needs of patients and their families. Ethical dilemmas arise in balancing the transition from curative to palliative care, respecting patient autonomy, and ensuring equitable access to services. Hospice care emphasizes beneficence (maximizing patient comfort), nonmaleficence (avoiding harm from unnecessary treatments), autonomy (informed decision-making), and justice (fair access to care), ensuring that patient care aligns with ethical and legal standards.

I

Immunization — Vaccine Hesitancy
Vaccine hesitancy refers to the reluctance or refusal to vaccinate despite the availability of vaccines, a challenge that affects public health, especially when healthcare providers exhibit hesitancy. Historical resistance to vaccines has evolved into contemporary concerns about safety, efficacy, and ethical issues. Among healthcare practitioners, vaccine hesitancy undermines public trust and patient safety. Ethical dilemmas arise when personal beliefs conflict with professional duties to promote health and prevent harm. Healthcare providers are ethically obligated to prioritize beneficence, nonmaleficence, and justice by advocating for immunization to protect patients and the broader community.

Impaired Drivers and Reporting
Reporting impaired drivers involves legal and ethical responsibilities for healthcare practitioners to ensure public safety while balancing patient confidentiality. Impairment can result from alcohol, medications, or medical conditions like epilepsy and dementia. Healthcare providers face ethical dilemmas between respecting patient autonomy and protecting public safety. Legal requirements for reporting impaired drivers vary by jurisdiction, and mandatory reporting may strain the patient-provider relationship. Practitioners must prioritize beneficence and nonmaleficence by preventing harm, ensuring fair application of reporting laws (justice), and maintaining clear communication with patients about the potential consequences of their health conditions on driving abilities.

Impaired Practitioners — Reporting
Reporting impaired practitioners is a crucial responsibility in healthcare, balancing patient safety with the rights and privacy of healthcare workers. Historically, the stigma around addiction or mental health issues in healthcare created silence around reporting. Today, healthcare practitioners face ethical dilemmas, such as the conflict between loyalty to colleagues and the duty to protect patients. Legal obligations vary by jurisdiction, but reporting is often mandated to prevent harm. Ethical principles like nonmaleficence and justice guide the need to ensure impaired practitioners receive help while prioritizing patient safety and maintaining public trust in the healthcare system.

Informed Consent
Informed consent is a fundamental ethical and legal requirement in healthcare, ensuring that patients or their surrogates have the ability to make voluntary and informed decisions about their medical care. For informed consent to be valid, several conditions must be met: the patient or surrogate must have decisional capacity to understand and make choices about their care; they must be fully informed of their diagnosis and prognosis, available treatment

options (including no treatment), and the benefits and risks associated with each option. The decision must be made without coercion, aligning with the patient's reasonable goals, values, and priorities. Finally, the decision must be communicated, documented in medical records, and shared with all relevant healthcare team members to ensure cohesive and ethical care

Interrogation — Healthcare Boundaries

Healthcare professionals' involvement in interrogations has been historically contentious, particularly regarding ethical standards in wartime and conflict. The Nuremberg Code, developed after World War II, set clear ethical guidelines prohibiting healthcare professionals from participating in coercive interrogations, which often involve physical or psychological harm. Contemporary dilemmas include balancing legal pressures with ethical duties to "do no harm." Professionals must uphold patient autonomy, beneficence, nonmaleficence, and justice, avoiding complicity in practices that violate human rights and undermine medical ethics. Their role is to heal, not to harm, ensuring that care and respect for individuals remain paramount.

- *Cross-reference: Autonomy, Capacity, Surrogate Decision-Making, Youth Consent*

J

Justice

Justice refers to the ethical obligation of healthcare practitioners to ensure fairness in the delivery of care. To implement justice as fairness, practitioners must provide treatment options that are equitable, ensuring that all patients receive appropriate care based on their medical needs, without discrimination or bias. These options must adhere to medical standards of care, institutional policies, and legal mandates, ensuring that all patients are treated with respect and dignity. By upholding the principle of public justice, practitioners contribute to a healthcare system that is fair, just, and committed to the equal treatment of all individuals.

- *Cross-reference: Autonomy, Beneficence, Nonmaleficence, Structural Injustice in Healthcare, Resource Allocation*

K

Kantian Ethics

Kantian ethics, rooted in the philosophy of Immanuel Kant, is a deontological ethical theory that prioritizes the inherent morality of actions based on adherence to duty and universal moral laws. According to Kantian principles, actions are morally right if they conform to a universal maxim that can be consistently willed as a universal law. In medical ethics, this approach emphasizes the respect for patient autonomy, requiring healthcare professionals to act with honesty and respect, treating patients as ends in themselves rather than means to an end. Kantian ethics stresses that moral actions are determined by duty and the intrinsic worth of individuals, regardless of the consequences.

L

Lifelong Learning

Lifelong learning is the continuous process of acquiring and updating medical knowledge and skills throughout a healthcare professional's career. Historically, medical education evolved from apprenticeships to formalized, structured learning, underscoring the need for ongoing education. Today, lifelong learning is essential for staying current with advancements in medical science, technology, and evidence-based practices. It ensures that healthcare providers meet professional, legal, and ethical standards, aligning with the principles of beneficence, nonmaleficence, and patient autonomy. By engaging in continuing education, practitioners can provide informed, high-quality care, ensuring that patient outcomes improve and healthcare standards are consistently maintained.

Living Will

A living will is a legal document that allows individuals to specify their preferences for medical treatment and end-of-life care in advance, in the event that they become incapacitated or unable to communicate their wishes. It typically outlines instructions regarding life-sustaining measures, such as the use of ventilators, feeding tubes, resuscitation efforts, and other interventions. By providing clear directives, a living will helps ensure that healthcare decisions align with the individual's values, beliefs, and desires, reducing uncertainty for family members and healthcare providers. It is an essential component of advance care planning, promoting patient autonomy and informed decision-making.

- *Cross-reference: Advance Directive, Durable Power of Attorney (DPOA), Patient Autonomy, End-of-Life Care*

M

Malpractice — Medical

Medical malpractice refers to a healthcare professional's failure to meet the accepted standard of care, resulting in harm to a patient. This concept dates back to ancient civilizations, with modern definitions shaped by legal and ethical guidelines. Key elements of malpractice include duty, breach of duty, causation, and damages. Malpractice cases arise from failures in communication, inadequate informed consent, or medical negligence. Ethical principles such as beneficence, nonmaleficence, and justice guide practitioners in avoiding malpractice by ensuring they act in the patient's best interest, minimize harm, and provide care that aligns with professional standards and patient rights.

Media Communications

Media communications in healthcare have historically been vital for public health campaigns, from early 20th-century efforts combating diseases like polio to modern digital health updates. While media enables widespread dissemination of information, ethical dilemmas arise regarding accuracy, potential public panic, and the balance between transparency and confidentiality. In today's digital age, misinformation can rapidly affect public trust and health behaviors, highlighting the need for responsible, evidence-based communication. Healthcare providers must adhere to ethical principles of autonomy, beneficence, and nonmaleficence, ensuring patient privacy is respected while providing clear, beneficial, and harm-free public health information.

Mediation

Mediation is a structured, voluntary process in which a neutral third party, known as the mediator, facilitates communication and negotiation between disputing parties to help them reach a mutually acceptable resolution. Unlike arbitration or litigation, mediation does not involve imposing a decision; instead, the mediator assists the parties in exploring their interests, identifying common ground, and developing solutions that satisfy both sides. Mediation is commonly used in various settings, including healthcare, family disputes, workplace conflicts, and legal cases, to resolve conflicts efficiently and amicably while preserving relationships and allowing parties to maintain control over the outcome.

Medical Records

Medical records are vital documents that track a patient's health history and treatments. Historically, they were controlled solely by healthcare providers, but evolving patient rights movements, particularly with the Health Insurance Portability and Accountability Act (HIPAA) in 1996, have shifted focus to patient autonomy. HIPAA ensures patients' right to access and control their Protected Health Information (PHI) while maintaining strict confidentiality. While Electronic Health Records (EHRs) enhance accessibility, they also raise concerns about privacy breaches. Balancing easy access to medical records with stringent privacy measures is crucial for upholding legal and ethical responsibilities in healthcare.

Minor Patients

Minor patients present unique ethical and legal challenges in healthcare. Historically, healthcare decisions were made by parents or guardians under the principle of *parens patriae*, with limited consideration of minors' autonomy. Over time, particularly in cases involving reproductive health and mental health care, minors' rights have expanded. Contemporary dilemmas involve balancing minors' autonomy with parental authority and legal mandates. While state laws vary, many allow minors to consent to certain types of care. Healthcare providers must respect minors' emerging autonomy, involve them in decision-making, and ensure care aligns with legal and ethical standards to prioritize their best interests.

N

Nonmaleficence

Nonmaleficence is the ethical principle requiring healthcare providers to avoid causing harm and to minimize the burdens on the patient. To uphold nonmaleficence, practitioners must offer treatment options that reduce potential physical, emotional, or psychological burdens, ensuring that these align with the patient's reasonable goals, values, and priorities. All treatment options presented must adhere to established medical standards of care, institutional policies, and legal mandates. By carefully selecting and managing treatment approaches, practitioners can prevent unnecessary suffering and safeguard the patient's well-being, consistently maintaining the commitment to do no harm.

- *Cross-reference: Beneficence, Justice, Autonomy, Weigh and Balance, Medical Harm*

Nurses and Allied Health Professionals
Nurses and allied health professionals have historically been viewed as supporting roles within a physician-led healthcare system. Over time, their roles have expanded, with many taking on greater decision-making responsibilities and providing direct patient care. Today, professionals such as nurse practitioners, physician assistants, and physical therapists are key to managing chronic conditions, preventive care, and patient education. This shift presents challenges related to scope of practice, interprofessional collaboration, and professional autonomy. These healthcare providers must navigate complex ethical, legal, and institutional frameworks to ensure patient care aligns with beneficence, nonmaleficence, autonomy, and justice.

O

Organ Donations
Organ donation has evolved significantly since the first successful transplant in 1954, transforming from a rare procedure to a vital part of modern healthcare. Ethical concerns include informed consent, the allocation of scarce organs, and the determination of death. Contemporary dilemmas involve balancing donor autonomy with public health needs, addressing disparities in organ availability, and ensuring fair access to transplants. Federal laws such as the National Organ Transplant Act (NOTA) and the Uniform Anatomical Gift Act (UAGA) provide legal frameworks to safeguard donors and recipients. Ethical considerations focus on maximizing benefits while minimizing harm and ensuring justice in the distribution of organs.

Organizational Ethics
Organizational ethics refers to the principles, values, and standards that guide the behavior and decision-making processes within an

organization. It encompasses the moral responsibilities of the organization toward its stakeholders, including employees, customers, suppliers, and the broader community. Organizational ethics involves establishing codes of conduct, ethical guidelines, and policies that promote integrity, accountability, fairness, and transparency. It also includes the creation of ethical cultures and frameworks to address ethical dilemmas, compliance with laws and regulations, and the promotion of ethical leadership. The goal is to ensure that all organizational activities align with ethical principles and contribute positively to society.

P

Palliative Care

Palliative care focuses on relieving suffering and improving the quality of life for patients with serious illnesses, integrating medical care with emotional, social, and spiritual support. Historically, healthcare emphasized life-prolonging treatments, often compromising patient comfort. The hospice movement led to the development of palliative care, advocating for a patient-centered approach that honors individual goals and values. Contemporary dilemmas include the timing of palliative care introduction, misconceptions about its role, and disparities in access. Legal frameworks such as the Patient Self-Determination Act (PSDA) ensure patient autonomy, while ethical principles emphasize maximizing benefits, minimizing harm, and ensuring equitable care for all patients.

Patient-Practitioner Relationship

The patient-practitioner relationship has shifted from a historically paternalistic approach, where practitioners made decisions without patient input, to a more collaborative model emphasizing patient autonomy. This shift, driven by the rise of patient-centered care, prioritizes shared decision-making, ensuring that care aligns with the patient's reasonable goals, values, and priorities. Ethical challenges arise in balancing practitioner expertise with patient autonomy, particularly with advancements in digital health and telemedicine. Ensuring trust, clear communication, and respect for patient rights remains critical. Legal frameworks, such as informed consent laws, support this relationship by safeguarding patient autonomy while ensuring practitioners act beneficently and minimize harm.

Practitioner Disagreements

Practitioner disagreements arise from differences in medical judgment, training, or interpretations of evidence-based practices. Historically, these were often resolved hierarchically, with senior practitioners making the final decisions. Modern interdisciplinary care, however, emphasizes collaborative resolution, respecting patient autonomy and promoting patient-centered outcomes. Unresolved disagreements can lead to confusion, delayed care, and potential harm, violating the principle of nonmaleficence. To resolve conflicts effectively, practitioners must balance ethical principles: autonomy (informed consent), beneficence (acting in the patient's best interest), nonmaleficence (avoiding harm), and justice (ensuring fairness in care). Structured conflict resolution processes help ensure optimal patient outcomes.

Precision Medicine

Precision medicine involves tailoring medical treatment to individual patient characteristics, such as genetic makeup, lifestyle, and environment. Unlike the traditional one-size-fits-all approach, it seeks to optimize patient care by personalizing therapies. While this innovative practice enhances Practitioner Beneficence by maximizing patient benefits, it also raises ethical concerns. These include Patient Autonomy (ensuring informed consent, especially regarding genetic testing implications), Practitioner Nonmaleficence (minimizing harm through responsible data use), and Public Justice (ensuring equitable access to precision medicine across diverse populations). Precision medicine offers great potential, but practitioners must balance its benefits with ethical obligations to ensure fair, individualized care.

Pregnant Patients
The treatment of pregnant patients historically prioritized paternalistic decision-making, often neglecting Patient Autonomy. Contemporary practice focuses on respecting pregnant patients' rights to make informed decisions about their healthcare, balancing maternal and fetal well-being. Ethical dilemmas arise when maternal and fetal interests conflict, with principles like Practitioner Beneficence and Nonmaleficence guiding care decisions. Legal frameworks, such as the Pregnancy Discrimination Act, protect pregnant patients from unfair treatment, ensuring equitable access to care under Public Justice. Healthcare providers must respect autonomy, provide patient-centered care, minimize harm, and ensure fairness in treating both the mother and fetus.

Preventive Ethics
Preventive ethics refers to proactive measures and strategies designed to identify, address, and mitigate potential ethical issues before they arise in healthcare and other professional settings. This approach focuses on preventing ethical dilemmas by implementing policies, training programs, and frameworks that guide decision-making and practice. Preventive ethics involves educating professionals about ethical principles, fostering a culture of ethical awareness, and establishing procedures for early intervention and resolution of ethical concerns. By addressing potential issues in advance, preventive ethics aims to enhance the quality of care, uphold ethical standards, and reduce the risk of ethical violations..

Product Sales in Healthcare
The sale of products to patients by healthcare providers raises ethical concerns related to conflicts of interest and patient trust. Historically, medical ethics emphasized a fiduciary duty, where physicians prioritized patient welfare over profit, and the introduction of direct sales risked undermining this principle.

Modern challenges include balancing Patient Autonomy by ensuring informed consent, while also adhering to Practitioner Beneficence, ensuring products benefit patients without compromising care. Legal frameworks like the Anti-Kickback Statute protect against financial exploitation. Providers must prioritize transparency and fairness (Public Justice) to avoid exploiting vulnerable populations, ensuring ethical, patient-centered care.

Protected Health Information (PHI)
Protected Health Information (PHI) refers to any information about an individual's health status, provision of healthcare, or payment for healthcare that can be used to identify the individual and is protected under privacy laws. PHI includes personal details such as names, addresses, dates of birth, Social Security numbers, medical records, and other health-related information. In the United States, PHI is safeguarded by the Health Insurance Portability and Accountability Act (HIPAA), which establishes standards for privacy and security to ensure that individuals' health information is kept confidential and secure from unauthorized access or disclosure.

Public Health Ethics
Public health ethics involves the moral considerations and principles guiding efforts to protect and promote the health of populations. Unlike clinical ethics, which focuses on individual patient care, public health ethics balances individual rights with collective well-being. Key ethical issues include ensuring fair access to healthcare resources, respecting autonomy while implementing public health measures (such as vaccination mandates and quarantine), and addressing health disparities. Public health initiatives must navigate the ethical tension between protecting individual freedoms and ensuring the common good, adhering to principles of justice, beneficence, nonmaleficence, and respect for autonomy.

- *Cross-reference: Justice, Autonomy, Vaccine Hesitancy, Confidentiality, Resource Allocation*

Q

Quality Improvement

Quality improvement (QI) is a systematic approach to enhancing the effectiveness, efficiency, and safety of healthcare services and processes. It involves continuous evaluation and refinement of practices based on data-driven analysis to achieve better patient outcomes and overall organizational performance. QI initiatives typically include setting specific goals, measuring performance against benchmarks, identifying areas for improvement, and implementing evidence-based changes. The process often involves multidisciplinary teams, feedback mechanisms, and iterative testing of interventions to ensure that improvements are sustainable and aligned with best practices and patient needs. By fostering a culture of continuous improvement, QI aims to enhance healthcare delivery and patient satisfaction.

R

Racial Concordance in Healthcare

Racial concordance refers to the practice of matching healthcare providers and patients based on race. Historically, it has been explored as a way to address racial disparities and improve patient satisfaction, particularly among minority populations. While racial concordance can foster better communication and trust, it does not necessarily guarantee higher-quality care. The ethical dilemma involves balancing patient autonomy—allowing patients to express racial preferences—with principles of justice and beneficence, ensuring all patients receive equitable, competent care. Ultimately, the goal is to build a healthcare system where racial concordance is unnecessary because all patients receive unbiased, high-quality care.

Referral and Fee Splitting in Healthcare
Referral and fee-splitting in healthcare, where providers receive compensation for referring patients, have raised ethical concerns historically and remain legally regulated. Fee-splitting can create conflicts of interest, compromising patient care and violating the principles of beneficence and nonmaleficence. Federal laws like the Stark Law and Anti-Kickback Statute prohibit such practices to protect patient autonomy and ensure referrals are based on clinical need, not financial gain. Ethically, providers must prioritize patient welfare, ensuring transparency in referrals and avoiding financial incentives that could undermine trust or create inequities in access to care.

Reportable Infections and Illnesses
Reportable infections and illnesses refer to certain diseases that healthcare providers must report to public health authorities to prevent and control outbreaks. Historically, this practice began with diseases like tuberculosis and cholera, but today it includes conditions like COVID-19, HIV, and measles. While essential for public safety, reporting can raise ethical tensions between protecting patient autonomy (privacy and consent) and fulfilling the duty of public justice (ensuring community health). Legal frameworks such as HIPAA provide exceptions for public health reporting, aiming to balance individual rights with the broader goal of beneficence and harm reduction in society.

Research and Clinical Equipoise
Clinical equipoise is the ethical principle that justifies conducting randomized controlled trials (RCTs) by ensuring there is genuine uncertainty in the medical community about which treatment is superior. Historically, it has safeguarded patient welfare by preventing the administration of knowingly inferior treatments. This concept aligns with the ethical principles of nonmaleficence

—ensuring no harm is done—and beneficence—aiming to maximize patient benefits. However, equipoise presents dilemmas when emerging evidence suggests one treatment's superiority, challenging researchers to uphold fairness (justice) and patient autonomy while ensuring that participants receive the best possible care based on evolving knowledge.

Research on Human Subjects

Research on human subjects involves ethical and legal considerations aimed at protecting participants' rights and welfare. Historical abuses, such as the Tuskegee Syphilis Study, led to the creation of key ethical guidelines, including the Nuremberg Code and the Belmont Report, which prioritize informed consent, beneficence, and justice. Federal regulations like the Common Rule mandate Institutional Review Board (IRB) oversight to ensure participant protection. The ethical challenge lies in balancing scientific progress with safeguarding individuals, ensuring that vulnerable populations are not exploited, and that research risks are minimized while potential benefits are maximized.

Resource Allocation

Resource allocation in healthcare refers to the ethical distribution of limited medical resources, such as organs, vaccines, or critical care beds, especially in times of scarcity. Ethical dilemmas arise in determining who should receive treatment first, balancing fairness, need, and the potential for benefit. Approaches to resource allocation often incorporate principles like justice (equitable access), beneficence (maximizing overall good), and nonmaleficence (minimizing harm). Decisions must consider both individual patient needs and the greater public health impact, ensuring transparency and fairness while avoiding discrimination and bias in the allocation process.

- *Cross-reference: Justice, Beneficence, Public Health Ethics, Triage Decision-Making, Ethical Decision-Making*

Root Cause Analysis (RCA):
Root Cause Analysis is a systematic process for identifying the underlying cause of adverse events in healthcare. In the context of biomedical ethics, it upholds the four principles: 1) Autonomy by ensuring patients' perspectives are considered; 2) Beneficence by promoting better outcomes through improved systems; 3) Nonmaleficence by minimizing harm by addressing root issues; and 4) Justice by ensuring equitable access to safer care. RCA helps healthcare teams improve patient safety and quality by addressing system flaws rather than blaming individuals.

S

Self, Family, and Friends Treatment
Treating oneself, family members, or friends presents significant ethical dilemmas due to the risk of compromised objectivity, confidentiality breaches, and conflicts of interest. Personal ties can cloud a physician's judgment, jeopardizing professional detachment needed to provide unbiased care. Ethical guidelines, such as those from the AMA, discourage this practice, emphasizing the potential harm to patient autonomy, beneficence, nonmaleficence, and public justice. Patients may withhold sensitive information, and physicians may avoid necessary procedures, resulting in suboptimal care. To ensure fairness and uphold ethical standards, physicians are advised to avoid treating individuals with whom they share personal relationships.

Sexual Boundaries
Sexual relationships between healthcare practitioners and patients undermine professional ethics due to the inherent power imbalance and potential for exploitation. These relationships violate patient autonomy by compromising the patient's ability to make free and informed decisions, while also undermining practitioner beneficence, as emotional involvement skews clinical judgment.

Nonmaleficence is breached when personal relationships result in emotional harm or disrupted care, and justice is denied as personal biases lead to unequal treatment. Ethical guidelines from the AMA and ACP emphasize maintaining strict professional boundaries to protect patient welfare and ensure unbiased, equitable care.

Sexually Transmitted Infections (STIs)
Sexually transmitted infections (STIs) refer to infections transmitted through sexual contact, which may or may not present symptoms. Historically stigmatized, STIs are now addressed through public health measures like mandatory reporting and expedited partner therapy (EPT), designed to control their spread. These interventions raise ethical dilemmas by balancing patient autonomy, confidentiality, and public health. The term STI, preferred over sexually transmitted disease (STD), reduces stigma and reflects that many infections do not progress to symptomatic disease. Managing STIs requires navigating legal, ethical, and medical responsibilities to protect both individual rights and community health.

SOAP Notes
The SOAP Notes Template provides a structured approach for documenting ethics consultations in healthcare, focusing on the bioethical principles of autonomy, beneficence, nonmaleficence, and justice. It includes four sections: Subjective, capturing the patient's or surrogate's perspective on their medical condition, diagnosis, prognosis, and treatment options, including ethical considerations; Objective, recording clinical facts and ensuring they align with medical standards of care; Assessment, evaluating the ethical issues, summarizing the THINK and ASSESS steps, and applying the TAC analysis to each bioethical principle; and Plan, outlining the recommended course of action, communication strategies, and adherence to ethical, legal, and medical standards.

Social Media Boundaries in Healthcare
Social media in healthcare presents unique ethical challenges, requiring healthcare professionals to balance personal expression

with patient confidentiality and professional integrity. Historically, healthcare interactions were confined to private consultations, but social media blurs these boundaries. Key dilemmas involve protecting patient privacy under laws like HIPAA, avoiding the disclosure of identifiable health information, and maintaining professional distance. Healthcare providers must ensure that their online presence adheres to ethical guidelines, such as those outlined by the AMA, to protect patient trust, confidentiality, and fairness, while responsibly using social media to promote public health.

Stages of Grief

The stages of grief, introduced by psychiatrist Elisabeth Kübler-Ross, outline the emotional responses individuals may experience when coping with significant loss or change. These stages include denial (initial shock and disbelief), anger (frustration and resentment), bargaining (attempts to reverse or mitigate the loss), depression (deep sadness and withdrawal), and acceptance (coming to terms with the loss and finding a way to move forward). While not necessarily experienced sequentially or by everyone, this model provides a framework for understanding the complex and personal process of grieving, recognizing that each individual's experience is unique.

Sterilization in Healthcare

Sterilization in healthcare, a permanent method of contraception, presents significant ethical concerns due to its historical misuse and the complexity of ensuring informed consent. Historically, involuntary sterilizations were performed on marginalized populations, leading to human rights violations. Today, sterilization must be voluntary, with a focus on protecting patient autonomy and preventing coercion. Ethical dilemmas persist around ensuring that patients fully understand the procedure's consequences, particularly for vulnerable groups. Balancing patient rights, informed consent, and equitable access to sterilization is essential for upholding the principles of autonomy, beneficence, nonmaleficence, and justice.

Strikes and Unionization in Healthcare
Strikes and unionization in healthcare present ethical dilemmas, as they balance healthcare workers' rights with the duty to ensure patient care. Historically, healthcare unions have advocated for better working conditions and patient care standards. However, strikes raise concerns about disrupting essential services, impacting patient well-being. Ethical challenges revolve around upholding patient autonomy, minimizing harm (nonmaleficence), promoting patient welfare (beneficence), and ensuring fairness (justice). While labor laws protect workers' rights to unionize, healthcare professionals must carefully manage strikes to ensure patients receive necessary care, adhering to bioethical principles to maintain patient trust and public health.

Structural Injustice in Healthcare
Structural injustice in healthcare refers to the systemic inequalities that lead to disparities in access, treatment, and outcomes for marginalized populations. Historically rooted in discriminatory practices such as racial segregation and biases in medical care, these injustices persist in modern healthcare. Examples include the Tuskegee Syphilis Study and ongoing disparities in maternal mortality among African American women. Addressing structural injustice requires healthcare providers to ensure equitable access, culturally competent care, and the dismantling of systemic barriers that perpetuate inequality. Ethical principles such as autonomy, beneficence, nonmaleficence, and justice guide efforts to rectify these long-standing inequities.

Student Involvement in Patient Care
Student involvement in patient care is a crucial component of medical education, offering students hands-on clinical experience under supervision. However, this practice raises ethical concerns, particularly regarding patient autonomy and informed consent.

Patients must be fully informed about the role of students in their care and provide explicit consent. Ethical principles like beneficence and nonmaleficence require careful supervision to ensure patient safety and quality of care, while justice demands that patients are treated equitably, regardless of their participation in student education. Balancing educational needs with patient rights is essential to uphold ethical standards in healthcare.

Substituted Judgment
Substituted judgment is a principle in surrogate decision-making where a surrogate makes healthcare decisions based on what the patient would have chosen, rather than their own preferences. The surrogate must align their decisions with the patient's reasonable goals, values, and priorities, all within the boundaries of medical standards of care, institutional policies, and legal requirements. This is a positive right of the patient, ensuring their autonomy is respected even when they cannot make decisions themselves. When properly followed, substituted judgment is protected by a negative right, meaning others cannot interfere with the surrogate's decision.

Surrogate Decision-Making
Surrogate decision-making occurs when a designated individual makes healthcare decisions on behalf of a patient who is unable to do so. This practice is grounded in patient autonomy, with surrogates expected to use substituted judgment—making decisions based on what the patient would have chosen, aligned with their reasonable goals, values, and priorities. Ethical challenges arise when surrogates' beliefs conflict with the patient's preferences. Surrogates must act within medical standards, institutional policies, and legal mandates. Effective surrogate decision-making balances patient autonomy, beneficence, nonmaleficence, and justice, ensuring care that reflects the patient's best interests.

- *Cross-reference: Substituted Judgment, Advance Directive, Durable Power of Attorney (DPOA), Patient Autonomy*

T

Telemedicine

Telemedicine leverages technology to deliver remote healthcare services, improving access for underserved and geographically isolated populations. While initially constrained by technology and cost, advancements have expanded its capabilities, offering real-time consultations and remote monitoring. However, telemedicine raises ethical dilemmas related to patient privacy, security, and the quality of care, particularly in the absence of physical exams. Federal regulations, such as HIPAA, ensure patient confidentiality, while telemedicine must align with patient autonomy, beneficence, nonmaleficence, and justice. Ensuring informed consent, safeguarding patient data, and addressing disparities in access are critical to ethically delivering telemedicine services.

Terminal and Palliative Sedation

Terminal or palliative sedation is used in end-of-life care to relieve intractable suffering by reducing a patient's consciousness without hastening death. Unlike euthanasia, its goal is to alleviate symptoms, not to shorten life. Ethical dilemmas arise regarding the balance between reducing suffering and the potential for life-shortening effects. Informed consent is crucial, ensuring patients or surrogates understand the permanent implications of sedation. Guided by the principles of autonomy, beneficence, nonmaleficence, and justice, terminal sedation is considered an ethically appropriate intervention when aligned with a patient's values and reasonable goals.

Testimonials and Avoiding Quackery

Testimonials have historically been used to promote unproven treatments, often leading to quackery, where claims are made without scientific validation. This practice raises significant ethical concerns about patient safety, informed consent, and the potential for misleading information. Modern ethical standards emphasize the need for transparency, requiring that testimonials used in healthcare be evidence-based and not mislead patients. Both the AMA and ACP stress the importance of promoting beneficence, nonmaleficence, and justice in healthcare marketing, ensuring that testimonials do not compromise patient autonomy or promote harmful, unproven therapies.

Torture and Enhanced Interrogation
Torture and enhanced interrogation involve coercive techniques, such as waterboarding and sleep deprivation, often used under the guise of extracting critical information, especially in military and political contexts. These practices have sparked global ethical, legal, and human rights debates, particularly regarding the balance between national security and human dignity. International law, including the United Nations Convention Against Torture (UNCAT), and U.S. legal protections like the Eighth Amendment, explicitly prohibit such methods. Ethical medical guidelines from organizations such as the AMA emphasize that healthcare professionals must not participate in or condone any form of torture or inhumane treatment.

Triage Decision-Making
Triage decision-making involves prioritizing patients based on the severity of their condition, particularly during emergencies when resources are limited. Originating in military medicine, triage aims to maximize survival by allocating care to those most likely to benefit. Contemporary dilemmas arise in balancing fairness, patient autonomy, and the ethical distribution of care, especially during crises like pandemics or disasters. Triage protocols must align with principles of beneficence, nonmaleficence, justice, and informed consent. Ensuring equitable access and transparency in decision-making is vital to maintaining trust in healthcare systems and upholding ethical standards.

U

Unemancipated Minor
An unemancipated minor is an individual under the age of legal adulthood who has not been granted legal independence from their parents or guardians. In most jurisdictions, this means the minor is still under the care and control of their parents or guardians, who are responsible for making legal, medical, and financial decisions on their behalf. The rights and responsibilities of unemancipated minors vary by jurisdiction but generally include limitations on their ability to consent to medical treatments, enter into contracts, or make other significant legal decisions without parental or guardian approval

Utilitarian Ethics
Utilitarian ethics is a normative ethical theory that evaluates the moral worth of actions based on their outcomes or consequences. Founded by philosophers such as Jeremy Bentham and John Stuart Mill, this theory posits that the best action is the one that maximizes overall happiness or well-being and minimizes suffering. Utilitarianism advocates for making decisions that produce the greatest good for the greatest number of people. This consequentialist approach focuses on the results of actions rather than the intentions behind them or adherence to rules, emphasizing efficiency and overall impact in moral decision-making.

V

Virtue Ethics
Virtue ethics is an ethical theory that emphasizes the role of character and virtue in moral decision-making, rather than focusing solely on the consequences of actions or adherence to rules. Rooted in the philosophy of Aristotle, virtue ethics asserts that moral behavior arises from cultivating virtuous traits such as

courage, temperance, and wisdom. According to this theory, a virtuous person acts in ways that align with these moral virtues, leading to a flourishing and fulfilling life. Unlike deontological or consequentialist approaches, virtue ethics prioritizes the development of moral character and the intention behind actions, aiming for the enhancement of individual and communal well-being.

W

Weigh and Balance
The Weigh and Balance process in ethical decision-making involves both the patient or surrogate and the practitioner collaboratively assessing the relative importance of the four primary bioethical principles: autonomy, beneficence, nonmaleficence, and justice. In the Weigh phase, they determine the weight of each principle based on the patient's reasonable goals, values, and priorities, while also considering medical standards of care, institutional policies, and legal mandates. In the Balance phase, they decide which principle or combination of principles should guide the decision-making process, aiming to arrive at a rational and reasonable recommendation that aligns with the patient's best interests and ethical obligations.

Withholding and Withdrawing Treatment
Withholding and withdrawing treatment refers to the ethical decision-making process of stopping or not initiating medical interventions when they no longer benefit the patient. Historically, medical ethics emphasized life preservation, but advancements in healthcare have raised dilemmas about when to forgo treatment that may prolong suffering. Contemporary practices prioritize patient autonomy, allowing individuals to refuse life-sustaining measures. Legal frameworks like the Patient Self-Determination Act (PSDA) support patient rights in these decisions. Balancing

autonomy, beneficence, nonmaleficence, and justice ensures that care aligns with patients' values while preventing unnecessary harm.

X

Xenotransplantation

Xenotransplantation refers to the transplantation of organs, tissues, or cells from one species to another, such as from animals to humans. This field raises significant ethical concerns, including issues of animal welfare, the potential for cross-species disease transmission, and the long-term implications for human health. Ethical debates focus on the justification for using animals in research and the possible impact on their well-being, as well as the need for rigorous safety testing and informed consent from patients who may receive xenotransplants. Additionally, considerations around the equitable distribution of such advanced treatments and their accessibility in different healthcare settings are central to the ethical discourse.

Y

Youth Consent:

Youth consent involves the ethical and legal considerations surrounding the ability of minors to make informed decisions about their own medical care and treatment. In many jurisdictions, minors are considered legally unable to provide consent for certain medical procedures, requiring parental or guardian approval. However, exceptions exist for specific situations, such as emergency care or certain types of confidential services like reproductive health. The concept of the "mature minor doctrine" applies in some cases, allowing minors deemed mature enough to consent to their own care. Ethical issues include balancing the respect for adolescent autonomy with the need for parental involvement, ensuring that minors understand their medical choices, and protecting their rights to make decisions that impact their health and well-being.

- *Cross-reference: Informed Consent, Capacity, Minor Patients, Confidentiality.*

Z

Zoonotic Diseases and Public Health

Zoonotic diseases, transmitted from animals to humans, have long impacted global health, with notable examples including the Black Death, rabies, and COVID-19. Historically, public health responses relied on quarantines and culling animals, raising ethical concerns about balancing human health, animal welfare, and environmental protection. Today, zoonotic diseases are exacerbated by urbanization and globalization, leading to ethical dilemmas regarding healthcare equity, resource allocation, and government mandates. Ethical responses to zoonotic outbreaks must balance autonomy, beneficence, nonmaleficence, and justice, ensuring fair and equitable access to healthcare while safeguarding public health.

- *Cross-reference: Public Health Ethics, Justice, Resource Allocction, Animal Welfare*

***

Author

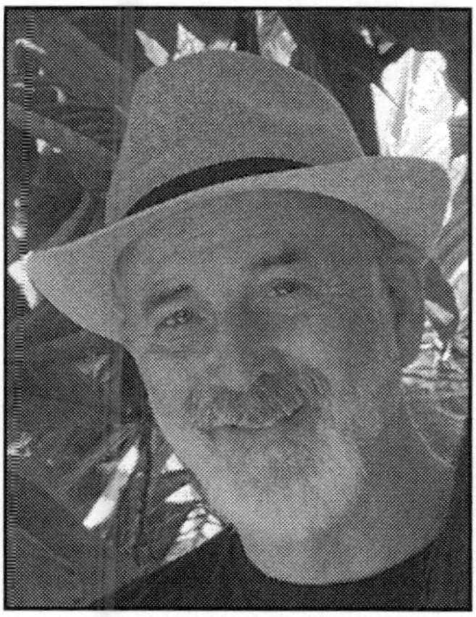

Dr. Jeffrey W. Bulger, PhD, has dedicated over 30 years to advancing bioethics consultation, policy development, and ethics education. He earned his PhD in Philosophy with a specialization in Medical Ethics from the University of Tennessee—Knoxville and was one of the first to be certified as a Healthcare Ethics Consultant (HEC-C). As Director of the Bioethics Program at The Chicago Medical School, Dr. Bulger has been instrumental in leading ethics consultations, developing ethical policies, and promoting ethics education within healthcare settings. His forthcoming book, *Bioethics: Passing the Boards, Providing Patient Care, and Beyond*, set to be published by Oxford University Press, reflects his continued dedication to integrating ethical principles into clinical practice.

In addition to his scholarly contributions, Dr. Bulger has chaired bioethics committees, mentored future leaders in the field, and advocated for the inclusion of bioethics in healthcare decision-making. He regularly engages in public and professional education, delivering presentations on a wide range of ethical topics. Dr. Bulger remains deeply committed to supporting the next generation of bioethics professionals, ensuring that ethical decision-making remains a cornerstone of patient care. His work continues to have a meaningful impact on shaping the ethical standards of healthcare today.

***